CONGESTIVE HEART FAILURE: SYMPTOMS, CAUSES AND TREATMENT

CARDIOLOGY RESEARCH AND CLINICAL DEVELOPMENTS

Focus on Atherosclerosis Research
Leon V. Clark (Editor)
2004. ISBN: 1-59454-044-6

Cholesterol in Atherosclerosis and Coronary Heart Disease
Jean P. Kovala (Editor)
2005. ISBN: 1-59454-302-X

Frontiers in Atherosclerosis Research
Karin F. Kepper (Editor)
2007. ISBN: 1-60021-371-5

Cardiac Arrhythmia Research Advances
Lynn A. Vespry (Editor)
2007. ISBN: 1-60021-794-X

Cardiac Arrhythmia Research Advances
Lynn A. Vespry (Editor)
2007. ISBN: 978-1-60692-539-3 (E-book)

Heart Disease in Women
Benjamin V. Lardner and Harrison R. Pennelton (Editors)
2009. ISBN: 978-1-60692-066-4

Heart Disease in Women
Benjamin V. Lardner and Harrison R. Pennelton (Editors)
2010. ISBN: 978-1-60741-090-4 (E-book)

Cardiomyopathies: Causes, Effects and Treatment
Peter H. Bruno and Matthew T. Giordano (Editors)
2009. ISBN: 978-1-60692-193-7

Cardiomyopathies: Causes, Effects and Treatment
Peter H. Bruno and Matthew T. Giordano (Editors)
2009. ISBN: 978-1-60876-433-4 (E-book)

Transcatheter Coil Embolization of Visceral Arterial Aneurysms
Shigeo Takebayashi, Izumi Torimoto and Kiyotaka Imoto (Editors)
2009. ISBN: 978-1-60741-439-1

Transcatheter Coil Embolization of Visceral Arterial Aneurysms
Shigeo Takebayashi, Izumi Torimoto and Kiyotaka Imoto (Editors)
2009. ISBN: 978-1-978-1-60876-797-7 (E-book)

Heart Disease in Men
Alice B. Todd and Margo H. Mosley (Editors)
2009. ISBN: 978-1-60692-297-2

Angina Pectoris: Etiology, Pathogenesis and Treatment
Alice P. Gallos and Margaret L. Jones (Editors)
2009. ISBN: 978-1-60456-674-1

Coronary Artery Bypasses
Russell T. Hammond and James .B Alton (Editors)
2009. ISBN: 978-1-60741-064-5

Congenital Heart Defects: Etiology, Diagnosis and Treatment
Hiroto Nakamura (Editor)
2009. ISBN: 978-1-60692-559-1

Congenital Heart Defects: Etiology, Diagnosis and Treatment
Hiroto Nakamura (Editor)
2009. ISBN: 978-1-60876-434-1 (E-book)

Atherosclerosis: Understanding Pathogenesis and Challenge for Treatment
*Slavica Mitrovska, Silvana Jovanova Inge Matthiesen
and Christian Libermans*
2009. ISBN: 978-1-60692-677-2

Practical Rapid ECG Interpretation (PREI)
Abraham G. Kocheril and Ali A. Sovari
2009. ISBN: 978-1-60741-021-8

**Heart Transplantation: Indications and Contraindications,
Procedures and Complications**
Catherine T. Fleming (Editor)
2009. ISBN 978-1-60741-228-1

**Heart Transplantation: Indications and Contraindications,
Procedures and Complications**
Catherine T. Fleming (Editor)
2010. ISBN 978-1-60876-591-1 (E-book)

Heart Disease in Children
Marius D. Oliveira and William S. Copley (Editors)
2009. ISBN: 978-1-60741-504-6

Heart Disease in Children
Marius D. Oliveira and William S. Copley (Editors)
2009. ISBN: 978-1-61668-225-5 (E-book)

Handbook of Cardiovascular Research
Jorgen Brataas and Viggo Nanstveit (Editors)
2009. ISBN: 978-1-60741-792-7

Handbook of Cardiovascular Research
Jorgen Brataas and Viggo Nanstveit (Editors)
2009. ISBN: 978-1-60741-792-7

Myocardial Ischemia: Causes, Symptoms and Treatment
Dmitry Vukovic and Vladimir Kiyan (Editors)
2010. ISBN: 978-1-60876-610-9

Congestive Heart Failure: Symptoms, Causes and Treatment
Josias E. García and Victoro R. Wright (Editors)
2010. ISBN: 978-1-60876-677-2

**Abdominal Aortic Aneurysms: New Approaches
to Rupture Risk Assessment**
*Barry J. Doyle, David S. Molony, Michael T. Walsh
and Timothy M. McGloughlin*
2010. ISBN: 978-1-61668-312-2

Cardiac Rehabilitation in Women
Arzu Daşkapan
2010. ISBN: 978-1-61668-146-3

Cardiac Rehabilitation in Women
Arzu Daşkapan
2010. ISBN: 978-1-61668-398-6 (E-book)

Oxidative Stress: A Focus on Cardiovascular Disease Pathogensis
Bashir M. Matata and Maqsood M. Elahi
2010. ISBN: 978-1-61668-157-9

Oxidative Stress: A Focus on Cardiovascular Disease Pathogensis
Bashir M. Matata and Maqsood M. Elahi
2010. ISBN: 978-1-61668-359-7 (E-book)

CARDIOLOGY RESEARCH AND CLINICAL DEVELOPMENTS

CONGESTIVE HEART FAILURE: SYMPTOMS, CAUSES AND TREATMENT

JOSIAS E. GARCÍA
AND
VICTORO R. WRIGHT
EDITORS

Nova Science Publishers, Inc.
New York

NOTICE TO THE READER

The Publisher has taken reasonable care in the preparation of this book, but makes no expressed or implied warranty of any kind and assumes no responsibility for any errors or omissions. No liability is assumed for incidental or consequential damages in connection with or arising out of information contained in this book. The Publisher shall not be liable for any special, consequential, or exemplary damages resulting, in whole or in part, from the readers' use of, or reliance upon, this material.

Independent verification should be sought for any data, advice or recommendations contained in this book. In addition, no responsibility is assumed by the publisher for any injury and/or damage to persons or property arising from any methods, products, instructions, ideas or otherwise contained in this publication.

This publication is designed to provide accurate and authoritative information with regard to the subject matter covered herein. It is sold with the clear understanding that the Publisher is not engaged in rendering legal or any other professional services. If legal or any other expert assistance is required, the services of a competent person should be sought. FROM A DECLARATION OF PARTICIPANTS JOINTLY ADOPTED BY A COMMITTEE OF THE AMERICAN BAR ASSOCIATION AND A COMMITTEE OF PUBLISHERS.

LIBRARY OF CONGRESS CATALOGING-IN-PUBLICATION DATA

Congestive heart failure : symptoms, causes, and treatment / editors, Josias
E. Garcma and Victoro R. Wright.
    p. ; cm.
Includes bibliographical references and index.
  ISBN 978-1-60876-677-2 (hardcover)
  1. Congestive heart failure. I. Garcma, Josias E. II. Wright, Victoro R.
  [DNLM: 1. Heart Failure. WG 370 C7518 2010]
  RC685.C53C673 2010
  616.1'29--dc22
                        2009054154
Available upon request

Published by Nova Science Publishers, Inc. ✦ New York

CONTENTS

PREFACE

Congestive heart failure (CHF) is a disease that originates from an inadequacy of the heart to maintain blood circulation, resulting in congestion and edema in the body tissues. CHF affects about five million patients in the US alone and an estimated 23 million patients worldwide, and is the only cardiac disease that is growing in prevalence, due to both increasing survival rates of myocardial infarctions and ageing population. In this book, the authors aim to uncover the many hormonal influences on myocardial function and discuss possible aetiological mechanisms, diagnostic modalities and management strategies of the Takotsubo syndrome.

Chapter 1 - Frequent monitoring of lung fluid content has a key role in the diagnosis and treatment of CHF patients as the edema severity can rapidly deteriorate to cause acute respiratory distress. Practiced techniques are divided into invasive or non-invasive, with the former being impractical for regular monitoring due to patient discomfort but also due to arguably low accuracy. Non-invasive techniques consist of imaging modalities, which again cannot be used on a daily basis or at home due to considerations e.g. costs and radiation. The bio-impedance technique has been proposed for over four decades as an alternative to existing non-invasive techniques, as in principle, the lung fluids content has a large impact on the thoracic electrical impedance. In this chapter we provide a concise overview on the research done thus far for adopting the bio-impedance principles to the measurement of lung congestion, starting from the transthoracic measurement approach proposed in the late 1960s to the more sophisticated electrical-impedance-tomography spectroscopy employed in recent years. The limitations and advantages of the various approaches will be discussed. In the main part of the chapter, we will present a hybrid bio-impedance approach that has been extensively studied in our lab for a robust and reliable diagnosis and monitoring of CHF patients. The technical design of a monitoring system, and the mathematics incorporated in the estimation of the left and right lung impedance values will be described. The results of several clinical studies that were aimed at evaluating the hybrid system's feasibility in detection, classification, and monitoring of edemic patients will be given, and we will conclude by discussing the implications of the results on the realization of hybrid bio-impedance systems in the clinic and home environments for the treatment of CHF patients.

Chapter 2 - The randomized trials with implantable cardioverter defibrillators (ICDs) have demonstrated clear benefits for patients with cardiomyopathy and systolic dysfunction. These trials have also provided rich data sets from these patients and have identified management issues which need more study. The MADIT II study demonstrated that ICDs reduced all-cause mortality in patients with coronary disease and a low ejection fraction. Appropriate shocks in this study predicted heart failure; inappropriate shocks predicted an increase in all cause mortality. The SCD-Heft study demonstrated that ICDs reduced all-cause mortality in patients with ischemic and nonischemic cardiomyopathy. Patients receiving both appropriate and inappropriate ICD shocks had an increase in all-cause mortality compared to patients who did not receive shocks; the most common cause of this mortality was heart failure. These two large studies demonstrate that ICD shocks are associated with heart failure progression. This may represent the natural history of these diseases, or it may represent the effect of shocks on myocardial function and/or interactions among shocks, the sympathetic nervous system, and psychiatric disorders associated with ICD use. Management issues include a careful selection of patients for ICD implantation. Other than the COMPANION study, randomized trials in patients with nonischemic cardiomyopathy do not demonstrate much benefit for those patients if they are on optimal medical therapy. ICDs need careful programming to limit the number of shocks and/or the energy required per shock. Medical management is crucial and should include beta-blockers and angiotensin converting enzyme inhibitors. The benefits with amiodarone therapy remain unclear in these patients. Physicians need to pay close attention to psychiatric symptoms with counseling, medication, and possible referral to psychiatrists. Cardiologists should use a standardized protocol to thoroughly review both the ICD device and medical care when these patients have shocks. More studies are needed on the importance of the New York Heart Association (NYHA) functional classification, psychiatric syndromes, and anti-arrhythmic medication use in these patients to limit complications and increase survival.

Chapter 3 - Takotsubo cardiomyopathy, also called left ventricular apical ballooning syndrome or ampulla cardiomyopathy is a clinical entity first described by Dote *et al* in the Japanese population, particularly in post-menopausal women [1]. Since then, this unique type of reversible left ventricular dysfunction has been increasingly reported in the literature and has provoked intense debate regarding its aetiology, natural history, treatment and long-term outcome. Through improving our understanding of this modern cardiomyopathy, we hope to unlock the secrets of myocardial stunning and hibernation, in addition to how endogenous hormonal imbalances may affect and even "break" our hearts.

In this chapter, we aim to uncover the many hormonal influences on myocardial function and discuss possible aetiological mechanisms, diagnostic modalities and management strategies of the Takotsubo syndrome. Furthermore, we shall try to understand what this 'new' cardiomyopathy has to teach us in relation to the modern care and treatment of not only the cardiac patient, but all our patients.

Chapter 4 - The pathogenesis of heart failure is associated with oxidative stress from the generation of reactive oxygen and nitrogen species, which leads to cardiac injury and dysfunction through a variety of means. Yet outcomes of recent interventional studies assessing the utility of anti-oxidants in protecting from cardiovascular disease that can cause heart failure have been disappointing. As discussed here, the ideas behind those studies were perhaps naive and a simple approach of targeting oxidative stress with dietary anti-oxidants is unlikely to be beneficial. The source and nature of the oxidative stress needs to be taken into account in devising therapeutic strategies. Moreover, intracellular redox signaling, which is activated by oxidative stress, plays a key role in cellular protection, as well as tissue repair and regeneration. Consequently, stem cell based therapies for heart failure will need to be mindful of the dual nature of oxidative stress to be fully effective.

Chapter 5 - Calcium ion has been found to play critical roles regulating both the beating and the growth of the heart. Mathematical modeling and computational simulations are required for understanding the complex dynamics arising from the calcium signaling networks controlling the heart growth, which is critical for devising therapeutic drugs for the treatment of pathologic hypertrophy and heart failure. In this paper, we will report our newest results of simulating the relevant calcineurin-centered calcium signaling pathways under the hypertrophic stimulus of pressure overload. We will show how the dual roles of RCAN protein in cardiac hypertrophy under different hypertrophic stimuli can be explained by the complex interactions of multiple signaling pathways and indicate how this particular example can help us understand the mystery of specificity encoding in calcium signaling networks. We will also discuss how to push forward the realistic modeling of calcium signaling network in mammalian hearts and how it can benefit from the corresponding calcium signaling research in simpler organisms such as yeast.

Chapter 6 - Right ventricular (RV) function plays an important role in the clinical outcome of cardiac surgery. RV failure observed in the operating room is notable for the bulging and distention of the RV free wall. When it occurs in the intra-operative period, RV failure is associated with failure to wean from cardiopulmonary bypass and the need for massive inotropic and mechanical support. Insufficient protection for RV remains to be an important limitation in current cardioplegic technique, either antegrade or retrograde, particularly in the context of RV hypertrophy and coronary artery disease. The RV has shown to be a risk factor of postoperative early mortality of valve surgery, coronary surgery, cardiac transplantation and implantation of left ventricular assist device (LVAD).

Chapter 7 – Background: CHF is one of the most important cardiac disorders in the US with a high incidence and prevalence as well as increased number of hospitalizations, deaths and, subsequently, increased health care costs.

Design: Meta-analysis of studies assessing BNP as a prognostic indicator.

Methods: Our objective is to determine if discharge BNP is an independent predictor of mortality and rehospitalization in patients admitted with CHF exacerbation. Our personal archives, MEDLINE, and reference lists of retrieved articles were searched. Two reviewers checked the list of abstracts and then the full papers for eligible studies and extracted data independently. We have started our search with 954 articles out of which 82 were selected for more detailed review. Only five studies met the eligibility criteria for the final meta-analysis. Our inclusion criteria were: age more than 18 years, CHF diagnosed by Framingham or echo criteria, BNP assessment in the 24 hour period prior to discharge and a minimum follow up period of one month. The outcomes assessed were all cause mortality and rehospitalization. Only observational, prospective cohort studies published in English language were included. We excluded all randomized control trials (as different treatment of different groups will introduce an additional bias), case series, case reports, case control studies, as well as studies that did not indicate clear clinical end points. The quality of the studies was assessed using the QUADAS (Quality Assessment of Diagnostic Accuracy Studies) score. Statistical analyses were performed using the fixed effects model calculated with Stats Direct and results were expressed as relative risks (RR). Receiver Operating Characteristics (ROC) curves were prepared using Dr. ROC software. We have used the I square test to appreciate the heterogeneity of the combined studies.

Results: The RR of death or rehospitalization for the three BNP cutoffs used 250, 350 and 500 pg/ml were 3.87, 4.66 and 5.73 respectively. For the 250 and 350 BNP cutoffs the Area Under the Curve (AUC) was 0.82 and 0.80.

Conclusion: BNP level at discharge is a strong independent predictor of early readmission or death in patients hospitalized with CHF exacerbation. Prior to discharging those patients health care providers should not only assess for clinical stability but also for circulatory stability by checking discharge BNP.

Chapter 8 - Heart rate variability is analyzed in time-domain or in frequency-domain. Three different novel non-invasive techniques for analysis of heart rate variability (R-R interval (RRI)) for the screening of patients with Congestive Heart Failure (CHF) are investigated. The first method, which is a time-domain method, is based on the Statistical Signal Characterization (SSC) of the analytical signal that is generated using Hilbert transformation of the RRI data. The four SSC parameters are: amplitude mean, period mean, amplitude deviation and period deviation. These parameters and their maximum and minimum values are determined over sliding segments of 300-samples, 32-samples and 16-samples for both the instantaneous amplitudes and the instantaneous frequencies derived from the analytical signal of the RRI data. Data used in this work are drawn from MIT database. The trial data used for estimating of the classification factor consists of 15 CHF (patient) subjects and 18 Normal Sinus Rhythm (NSR) or simply normal subjects. The performance of the algorithm is then evaluated on test data set consists of 17 CHF subjects and 53 NSR subjects. This new technique correctly classifies 31/33 of trial data and 65/70 of test data

The second and third techniques, which are frequency-domain methods, are based on the soft-decision wavelet-decomposition algorithm for estimating an approximate power spectral density (PSD) of (RRI) of ECG data for screening of congestive heart failure (CHF) from normal subjects. In the second method, the ratio of the power in the low-frequency (LF) band to the power in the high-frequency (HF) band of the RRI signal is used as the classification factor. Results are shown for 9 different wavelets filters. This new technique shows a classification efficiency of 93.93% on trial data and 88.57% on test data. An FFT-based frequency domain screening technique is also implemented and included in this chapter for the purpose of comparison with the wavelet-based technique. The FFT-based technique shows an efficiency of classification of 93.93% on trial data and 81.42% on test data.

In the third technique, which is a pattern recognition technique, two standard patterns of the base-2 logarithmic values of the reciprocal of the approximate PSD of sub-bands resulted from wavelet decomposition of RRI data of CHF patients and normal subjects are derived by averaging all corresponding values of all sub-bands of 12 CHF data and 12 normal subjects in the trial set. The computed pattern of each data under test is then compared band-by-band with both standard patterns of CHF and normal subjects to find the closest pattern. This new simple technique results in 90% identification accuracy by applying it on the test data.

In: Congestive Heart Failure…
Editors: J. E. García et al. pp. 1-35

ISBN: 978-1-60876-677-2
© 2010 Nova Science Publishers, Inc.

Chapter 1

MONITORING PULMONARY EDEMA IN CHF PATIENTS WITH A HYBRID BIO-IMPEDANCE APPROACH

Sharon Zlochiver, Shimon Abboud and Marina Arad

Dept. of Biomedical Engineering, Tel Aviv University, Ramat Aviv, Israel

ABSTRACT

Frequent monitoring of lung fluid content has a key role in the diagnosis and treatment of CHF patients as the edema severity can rapidly deteriorate to cause acute respiratory distress. Practiced techniques are divided into invasive or non-invasive, with the former being impractical for regular monitoring due to patient discomfort but also due to arguably low accuracy. Non-invasive techniques consist of imaging modalities, which again cannot be used on a daily basis or at home due to considerations e.g. costs and radiation. The bio-impedance technique has been proposed for over four decades as an alternative to existing non-invasive techniques, as in principle, the lung fluids content has a large impact on the thoracic electrical impedance. In this chapter we provide a concise overview on the research done thus far for adopting the bio-impedance principles to the measurement of lung congestion, starting from the transthoracic measurement approach proposed in the late 1960s to the more sophisticated electrical-impedance-tomography spectroscopy employed in recent years. The limitations and advantages of the various approaches will be discussed. In the main part of the chapter, we will present a hybrid bio-impedance approach that has been extensively studied in our lab for a robust and reliable diagnosis and monitoring of CHF patients. The technical design of a monitoring system, and the mathematics incorporated in the estimation of the left and right lung impedance values will be described. The results of several clinical studies that were aimed at evaluating the hybrid system's feasibility in detection, classification, and monitoring of edemic patients will be given, and we will conclude by discussing the implications of the results on the realization of hybrid bio-impedance systems in the clinic and home environments for the treatment of CHF patients.

1. PULMONARY EDEMA IN CHF PATIENTS – ORIGINS AND MEASURING TECHNIQUES

Congestive heart failure (CHF) is a disease that originates from an inadequacy of the heart to maintain blood circulation, resulting in congestion and edema in the body tissues. Cardiogenic pulmonary edema (CPE) is a major cause of morbidity and mortality in CHF patients. The inability of the heart to pump blood in proportion to the tissues' metabolism results in a compensatory increase in pulmonary venous pressure. Once the hydrostatic pressure in pulmonary capillaries exceeds the plasma oncotic pressure, fluid and colloid start leaking through the alveolo-capillary membrane. Pulmonary congestion occurs when lymphatic outflow does not suffice to remove the fluid accumulating in the interstitium. As the intravascular pressure increases along with the amount of extravascular liquid, the lungs become less compliant and less permeable to oxygen, leading to respiratory discomfort (dyspnea), hypoxemia and tachypnea. As the condition deteriorates, the capacity of the interstitial space is exceeded, the fluid floods the alveoli and airways resulting in full-blown CPE, an acute respiratory distress and a major medical emergency in heart failure patients (Guyton 1991).

CHF affects about 5 million patients in the US alone and an estimated 23 million patients worldwide, and is the only cardiac disease that is growing in prevalence, due to both increasing survival rates of myocardial infarctions and ageing population (Hunt et al. 2001, AHA 2005 statistics). The disease causes substantial patient suffering, and timely diagnosis and treatment of pulmonary congestion is of a great importance, as CPE can rapidly deteriorate to respiratory insufficiency, further impair cardiac function, and prove fatal. Current monitoring techniques are divided into invasive or non-invasive techniques. The thermal dye double-indicator dilution is an invasive technique for monitoring lung fluids, which is complex to employ as a standard monitoring routine since it incorporates the insertion of two catheters. Moreover, it provides an accuracy of only about 20%, it underestimates congestion level in patients with intravascular pulmonary shunts, and is inaccurate in some cases such as asymmetrical lung fluid content (unilateral pulmonary congestion) or poorly perfused lung regions (Brown et al. 1996, Kunst et al. 1998). Non-invasive techniques include mainly imaging modalities, e.g. X-ray radiographs. Although widely practiced, the clinical diagnostic value of X-ray chest radiographs has been found to be inconsistent (Staub 1986, Chakko et al. 1991, Balbarini et al. 1991, Liebman et al. 1978), and the technique suffers from limitations due to interpretation difficulties caused by coexisting lung diseases (Gehlbach and Geppert 2004). Other imaging modalities e.g. CT, NMR or MRI, demonstrate high accuracy of as much as ~3%, however involve either ionizing radiation or large expenses that preclude them from frequent utilization (Patroniti et al. 2005, Hayes et al. 1982). Weighing is also commonly employed for monitoring PE, though it is obviously not a specific indicator to the lung fluids amount. Therefore, it is beneficial to have an alternative method that is capable of monitoring PE in CHF patients.

2. THE BIO-IMPEDANCE APPROACH IN MEASURING PULMONARY EDEMA

The electrical properties of edemic lungs are considerably different from those of healthy lungs due to the change in the proportion of fluids and air, which is much higher in the former case. As lung fluids are characterized by a lower impedivity than air, monitoring the development of lungs' impedivity is expected to indicate their amount. The bio-impedance technique retrieves information regarding the electrical properties of inner-tissues by measuring the developing voltage due to applied electrical current. It can be operated non-invasively by attaching electrodes to the body surface, from which low-amplitude, low-frequency current is injected and voltages are measured. Typically, the current frequency is set to $O(10^4 Hz)$, low enough for minimizing the capacitive effects of the tissues, yet high enough to meet safety requirements. Currently, there are two approaches in adapting the bio-impedance principles for PE monitoring. The transthoracic measurement approach was the first to be suggested in the late 60s (Pomeranz et al. 1969), and since then it was extensively developed and improved by many others (Fein et al. 1979, Saunders 1988, Zellner et al. 1990, Charach et al. 2001). The method is based on the measurement of the voltage between two electrodes, attached to the patient's neck and waist, as current is injected via another pair of electrodes, attached in proximity to the measuring electrodes. The second, newer approach is based on a technology called electrical impedance tomography (EIT), which was first introduced in the mid 80s (Brown et al. 1985). Thoracic EIT involves the attachment of an electrode array around the thorax and the successive current injections, each via a different electrode pair, and the simultaneous voltage measurement via the remaining electrodes. By employing sophisticated reconstruction algorithms, EIT is capable of retrieving an axial image of the inner-thoracic impedivity spatial distribution. Usually 16 or more electrodes in the array are employed for retrieving acceptable image resolution, though the achievable resolution is still much lower than what can be retrieved by other imaging modalities. In the mid 80s the use of EIT for monitoring pulmonary functions, among them CPE, was suggested by Harris et al. (Harris et al. 1987, Harris et al. 1988). They predicted that a change in the lung-fluid amount of about 10ml should be measurable by EIT system. Newell et al. induced pulmonary edema in six Mongrel dogs by means of injecting oleic acid (Newell et al. 1996). A 32-electrodes real-time EIT system (ACT3) and a fast NOSER algorithm were used to reconstruct admittivity images of the thorax during the experiment. An increase in the lungs' conductivity of $4–6mSm-1$, and a clear correlation between the edema development and the reconstructed conductivity change were found. Frerichs et al. used a 16-electrode EIT system to measure pulmonary edema induced by injection of oleic acid into the left lung of five pigs, and succeeded in detecting the local, unilateral lung damage using EIT imaging (Frerichs et al. 1998). Human studies were performed for several related clinical conditions: normal subjects undergoing intravenous infusion (Campbell et al. 1994a, Campbell et al. 1994b), normal patients undergoing changes in lung fluids induced by diuretics (Noble et al. 2000), emphysema patients with a variable degree of lung parenchyma destruction (Kunst et al. 1998), and patients suffering from pulmonary edema due to non-cardiogenic acute respiratory failure and congestive heart failure (Kunst et al. 1999). Most of these studies used the Sheffield (Mark 1 or Mark 3) hardware with a back-projection reconstruction algorithm and showed that EIT can detect the resistivity (or conductivity) changes associated with the change in the lungs' fluids content. In another approach, EIT spectroscopy, where impedance data is collected at several frequencies, can be employed for monitoring lung resistivity changes. Brown et al. measured maturational changes in lung resistivity spectra on a group of children aged between birth and 3 years old (Brown et al. 2002). An eight-electrode EIT system (Sheffield Mark 3.5) was used with 30 excitation frequencies, and the data was calibrated and parametrically fitted to a Cole model for the lung tissue. A good agreement between the reconstructed lung resistivity spectra and the expected spectra from theoretical models was found. Both bio-impedance approaches (i.e., the transthoracic measurement and EIT) present some attractive technical benefits over other PE monitoring methods: 1) the technique is safe, utilizing only very small amplitude AC currents, without the use of ionizing radiation or strong magnetic fields; 2) data can be collected continuously and over long-term periods, providing temporal information; and 3) the hardware is relatively easy to construct in a low cost and the system can be designed to be portable. Nevertheless, the bioimpedance technique exhibits also a functional benefit, as it provides a unique physical quantity (tissue's impedivity), which no other monitoring technique or imaging modality can retrieve, and which in many medical cases can indicate a pathology (Holder 1993). On the other hand, each of the bio-impedance approaches bears its characteristic disadvantages. An inherent limitation of the transthoracic impedance approach is that it cannot directly specify the impedivity of the thoracic internal organs, e.g. the lungs in the case of PE monitoring. Moreover, it is largely dependent on the anthropometric parameters of the patient and has not been shown to provide consistent results so far (Noble et al. 1999). While EIT overcomes this limitation by solving for the spatial impedivity distribution, it has major technical limitations, mainly due to the requirement to attach a large number of electrodes to the patient's thorax. In addition, it is highly sensitive to measurement noise, either due to electrical noise on the electrodes or uncertainty regarding the precise electrodes' locations (Jongschaap et al. 1994). Due to these limitations, EIT is currently employed mostly in research studies, using laboratory systems, and is not practiced in the clinics.

In this chapter we describe a portable bio-impedance system ("CardioInspect" Tel-Aviv University, Israel), which combines some of the features of both bio-impedance approaches, and that was designed and built for the medical application of CPE monitoring. The system consists of an eight-electrode belt, and rather than a full spatial impedivity distribution or a single transthoracic impedance value, it provides estimations for two parameters—the left and the right lung resistivity. In addition, the system measures the ECG signal, needed for synchronization of the bio-impedance measurement procedure, and provides complementary information essential for cardiogenic PE monitoring. This hybrid system is believed to improve the diagnostic capabilities of this illness, and help the physicians to better adjust the proper medication dosage on a frequent basis.

3. A HYBRID BIO-IMPEDANCE SYSTEM FOR DIAGNOSING AND MONITORING CHF PATIENTS

3.1. Technical Design

3.1.1. Hardware design

A block diagram and a photograph of the experimental system are presented in Figure 1(a) and (b) respectively. The system comprises of an eight-electrode belt, worn around the thorax, with an additional reference electrode attached to the waist for minimizing baseline drifts. All nine electrodes are disposable Ag/AgCl electrodes. Each one of the eight units comprising the belt has five degrees of length, so that the belt can be adjusted to different thorax sizes (from 85 to 135cm), while ensuring evenly spaced locations of the electrodes. A current source circuit generates a sinusoidal current (3mA peak-to-peak, 20kHz), which is injected through a switch matrix to the body in an opposite configuration. For each injection, differential voltages are measured using the four-electrode method (Grimnes and Martinsen 2000) and amplified by a factor of 50 to a level of several volts. These voltages measurements are filtered using a band-pass filter (BPF) with a central frequency of 20kHz and a bandwidth of 1kHz, and sampled at $f_s =$ 250kHz in a resolution of 16 bits using an A/D chip (TI-ADS8323). The system also measures the ECG signal using two of the eight electrodes for a period of 5sec (electrodes 3 and 8 in Figure 2(a)—between the right and the left sides of the thorax). The ECG signal is filtered using a BPF in the range of 0.05–30Hz and sampled at $f_s = $ 1kHz. The measurement sequencing is controlled by a microprocessor (TMS320VC5416) and performed in the following order: a 5-sec long ECG signal is first measured and analyzed in real-time for extracting the mean RR interval. A delay of 1/3RR from the last detected R-wave is used as a trigger for the following bio-impedance measurements, so that all measurements are performed during the iso-potential interval of the cardiac cycle, in order to keep the shape and position of the heart as constant as possible. In addition, all measurements are performed during shallow tidal respiration and in the same sitting posture so that lungs' resistivity would not be affected largely by breathing. The entire measurement lasts less than 30sec. The system is powered by a rechargeable battery for complying with patient safety limitations, and has a measured signal-to-noise ratio of ~75 dB, calculated as the average ratio between the standard deviation and the mean of voltage measurements (Brown 1993).

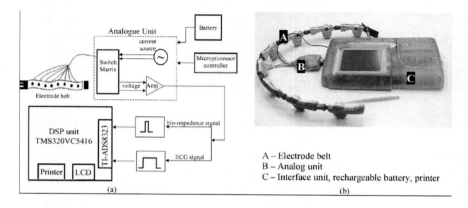

Figure 1. (a) Schematic diagram of the experimental system. (b) A photograph of the experimental system (Zlochiver et al. 2007, needs permission).

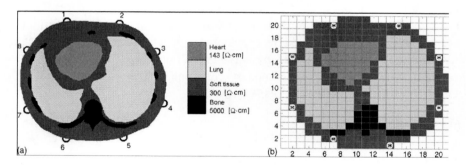

Figure 2. (a) The original two-dimensional thorax model, which was assumed constant in the inverse-problem solver. The positions of the eight electrodes and the resistivity values for the various tissues are marked. The left and right lung resistivity values are the two parameters to be optimized by the inverse-solver. (b) The low-resolution geometry model that was employed in the reconstruction algorithm (Zlochiver et al. 2007, needs permission).

3.1.2. Software design

Lung resistivity estimation

An iterative parameter optimization scheme, based on the second-order Newton–Raphson method (Yorkey et al. 1987), was implemented for estimating the left and right-lung resistivity values, each was assumed constant in its respective lobe domain. The method comprises of guessing an initial conductivity for each lung lobe, calculating the expected surface potentials due to the injected currents for all source and sink configurations, and comparing them to the respective measured surface voltages from the thoracic electrode belt. Then, at every iteration, new resistivity values for the two lungs are updated so that the error, defined by the Euclidean distance between the calculated and the measured surface potentials, is reduced, until a predefined stopping criterion is fulfilled. A constant two-dimensional thorax model was employed for all subjects in the inverse algorithm, where all tissue geometry and resistivity, except for the lungs' resistivity values, are regarded pre-known. In Figure 2(a), the original geometry model, based on an axial CT image, is shown after segmentation to four main tissues, along with the positions of the eight belt electrodes. Each of the tissues was assigned with an appropriate resistivity value taken from the literature (Gabriel et al. 1996) ($\rho_{heart} = 143\Omega$cm, $\rho_{soft\ tissue} = 300\Omega$cm, $\rho_{bone} = 5000\Omega$cm). A low-resolution (20x20) geometry model was employed for the reconstruction algorithm, shown in Figure 2(b). The surface potentials, which are needed during the iterative process, are calculated by solving the following governing Laplace equation with Neumann type boundary condition, which is an extension of Ohm's law (Morucci and Marsili 1996):

$$\nabla \cdot \left(\frac{1}{\rho}\nabla\varphi\right) = 0 \quad , \tag{1}$$

$$\frac{1}{\rho}\frac{\partial\varphi}{\partial\vec{n}} = \begin{cases} \vec{J}, & on\ electrode\ positions \\ 0, & elsewhere \end{cases} \tag{2}$$

where ρ (Ωm) is the tissue resistivity, φ (V) the electrical potential, $\vec{J}$ (A m^{-2}) the injected current density and $\vec{n}$ is a unit vector normal to the boundary. The boundary condition specifies that no current flow into the surrounding insulating air except at the locations of the injecting electrodes. In the physical model expressed by eqs. (1) and (2), several assumptions and simplifications were applied, including the quasi-static approximation and linearity and isotropy of the biological volume conductor. The finite-volume method was employed for the discretization and the numerical solution of the integral presentation of the governing equation by taking a surface integral on (1) and applying Gauss' divergence theorem:

$$\oint_l \frac{1}{\rho} \nabla \varphi \cdot d\vec{l} = 0$$

(3)

where $d\vec{l}$ (m) is a vector length element. As was previously mentioned, only the values of the lungs' resistivity are updated at every iteration, while the resistivity values and the geometrical shape of all other tissues are kept fixed. For the k'th iteration, the update is performed using the following formula (Yorkey et al. 1987):

$$\vec{\rho}_{k+1} = \vec{\rho}_k - \left(\mathbb{J}_k^T(\vec{\rho}_k) \mathbb{J}_k(\vec{\rho}_k) \right)^{-1} \mathbb{J}_k^T(\vec{\rho}_k)(\vec{\varphi}_s(\vec{\rho}_k) - \vec{\varphi}_0)$$

(4)

where $\vec{\rho}_k = \begin{bmatrix} \rho_{right} \\ \rho_{left} \end{bmatrix}$ is the lung resistivity parameter vector at the k'th iteration, $\vec{\varphi}_s(\vec{\rho}_k)$ is a concatenated vector of the surface potentials calculated for all current injections at the k'th iteration, $\vec{\varphi}_0$ is a similar concatenated vector containing the measured surface voltages, and $\mathbb{J}_k$ is the k'th iteration Jacobian matrix, defined as $\mathbb{J}_k = \partial\vec{\varphi}_s(\vec{\rho}_k) / \partial\vec{\rho}_k$. A comprehensive formulation of the numerical solution of (3) and (4) can be found in previous works (Radai et al. 1999a, Radai et al. 1999b, Zlochiver et al. 2004, Zlochiver et al. 2003). Although the inverse solver results are described as absolute resistivity values, they are in practice normalized by a scaling factor. This factor was calculated so that the average reconstructed lung resistivity for healthy, non-edemic subjects, was equal to the value known from the literature in tidal respiration (Wang and Patterson 1995) (ρnormal$\sim$=1100Ωcm at O(10 kHz)).

RR and QT interval calculation

An R-wave detection algorithm was applied on the 5sec-long ECG signal, which employed a BPF (8–30 Hz) to extract the QRS-complexes from the rest of the ECG and a threshold based peak-detection method to locate the peaks of the R-waves. Although the ECG was measured using two of the belt electrodes, thus providing a non-standard signal, the acquired signal still provided the temporal information required for extracting the RR and QT intervals. The ECG-signal beats were averaged using the detected R-wave peaks for synchronization, resulting in an average ECG beat. From the averaged beat, the QT interval, defined as the time from the beginning of the QRS-complex to the end of the T-wave, and which represents the total ventricular activity composed of the depolarization and repolarization periods, was measured (Figure 3). Finally, the corrected QT-RR, normalized to a heart-rate of 60 bpm, was calculated using Bazett's formula (Bazett 1920):

$$QT_c = {QT}/{\sqrt{RR}} \tag{5}$$

where QT_c (sec) is the corrected QT interval and RR (sec) is the mean time period between sequential R-waves.

3.2. Clinical Results

The following section presents a set of experimental trials that were conducted in order to assess the feasibility of the bio-impedance measurements to detect, classify and monitor CHF patients suffering from CPE.

3.2.1. Baseline measurements

A set of tests was conducted in order to evaluate the measurement performance of the hybrid bio-impedance system at baseline, i.e. for non-edemic subjects. A reproducibility test was performed on three healthy male subjects (aged 54, 39 and 32 years old). The subjects were measured three times in a 5-month period, with the electrode belt removed after each measurement session. Within each session, five consecutive measurements were taken, while keeping the electrode belt attached to the thorax. In Figure 4, the left and right lung-resistivity reconstructions are presented for the three subjects. The mean and standard deviation of the resistivity values are shown for the three measurement sessions. The results demonstrate a both within-test and between test reproducibility (i.e. with and without belt removal) of less than 2%.

Another study was conducted to check whether there was a dependence of lung resistivity reconstruction on anthropometric parameters. If such dependence were to be found, then the system would have had to be calibrated per patient's parameters. A sample of $N= 33$ healthy male subjects (50 ± 16 years old) was included for this study. A paired t-test was performed for studying the dependence of the mean reconstructed lung resistivity value on various anthropometric parameters—age, height, weight, body mass index (BMI) and body surface area (BSA). Table 1 summarizes the resulting correlations and p-values, from which it is clear that there was no dependency of the resistivity reconstructed values on any of the tested anthropometric parameters, implying that any possible difference in the resistivity values between the control group and the CHF group most likely originates from the pathologic condition.

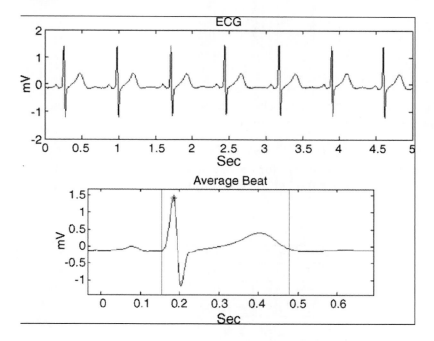

Figure 3. An example for a 5-s long ECG signal measured by the system (up) and the respective averaged beat with automatic markings of the QT interval (down), Zlochiver et al. 2007 (needs permission).

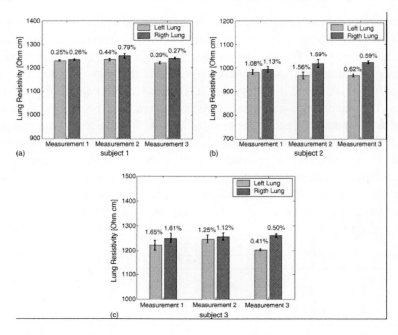

Figure 4. Reproducibility test results. (a) Subject 1; (b) subject 2; (c) subject 3. Zlochiver et al. 2007 (needs permission).

Table 1. *t*-Test summary for the dependence of the reconstructed lung resistivity values on various anthropometric parameters.

Parameter	R	p-Value
Age	0.26	0.18
Height	0.13	0.50
Weight	0.08	0.68
BMI	0.04	0.84
BSA	0.10	0.61

3.2.2. CHF patients' classification and long-term monitoring

A clinical study was initiated to test the capability of the bio-impedance system to classify and differentiate CHF patients with CPE from non-edemic subjects. The study was conducted at the CHF clinic of the Department of Cardiology, Rabin Medical Center in Israel, and was approved by a local Helsinki ethics committee. The inclusion criteria for subject participation in the study were: 1) absence of a cardiac implantable device; and 2) a signed informed consent form. The study was performed on two subject groups, the first of which was the control group of 33 healthy subjects studied in section 3.2.1, while the second group consisted of 34 male CHF patients (56 ± 13 years of age) with various degrees of CHF severity, regularly monitored at the clinic. An unpaired t-test was performed, showing no significant difference between the ages of the two study groups ($p \cong 0.12$). The reconstruction results for the lung resistivity values of the two study groups are shown in Figure 5. In this graph, the right lung vs. the left lung reconstructed resistivity values are plotted for all subjects. An apparent separation between the two groups was observed, wherein the CHF patients had lower lung resistivity values, indicating larger fluid volumes in the lungs. The mean left and right resistivity for the control group was 1205 ± 163 and 1200 ± 165 Ωcm and for the CHF group 888 ± 193 and 943 ± 187 Ωcm. An unpaired two-sample t-test proved this separation to be significant for both lungs (with $p < 2 \cdot 10^{-7}$). It was noticed that while the mean resistivity value for the left and right lungs was balanced for the control group, the right lung resistivity was larger by 55Ωcm than the left value for the CHF group, although not significantly ($p = 0.23$). The system capability for long-term monitoring of edema severity was tested on two CHF patients (aged 53 and 67 years for subjects 1 and 2, respectively). These patients were measured three times in a period of a few weeks while in medication treatment. The left and right lung resistivity reconstruction values for the two patients are shown in Figure 6 as a function of measurement in time. A general increase in both lung resistivity values was measured for both subjects, indicating an improvement in the edema severity level. This improvement was found to correlate with an expert physician diagnosis as well as with the decrease in weight for the two patients (from 72 to 64kg and from 63 to 60kg for subjects 1 and 2, respectively).

3.2.3. Monitoring CHF patients under intravenous diuretics treatment

As aforementioned, timely treatment of pulmonary congestion in CHF patients is of great importance, as CPE can rapidly deteriorate to respiratory insufficiency, further impair cardiac function and may even prove fatal. This is usually achieved by introducing diuretic agents, which remove excessive body fluids through the passing of urine. However, diuresis over-treatment can result in hypovolemia, thus reducing cardiac output, interfering with renal function and producing weakness and lethargy. Diuretics might also cause hypokalemia due to a concentration decrease of important ions in the blood circulation. Therefore, for optimizing medicinal treatment with diuretics, i.e., to allow accurate lung fluid management, one should be able to monitor temporal changes in the lungs' fluid content on a frequent basis (Schuller *et al* 1991). To address this challenge, we have studied the performance of the hybrid bio-impedance system with patients under diuretics treatment. A clinical study was conducted at the department of cardiology in Sheba Medical Center, Israel, and was approved by a local ethics committee. A study group consisted of 13 regularly monitored CHF patients (all males, aged 64 ± 9 years), all of whom signed an informed consent and were not carrying a cardiac pacemaker or other implantable device. Two bio-impedance measurements of the left- and right-lung resistivity were taken for each subject during diuretics treatment—one measurement before an intravenous injection of Fusid and one following a resting period of approximately 4 h. The medication dose was typically 80 (range 40–120) mg furosemide by intravenous drip. The main factors determining the diuretic dose in these adult CHF patients were the extent of volume overload, renal function and prior responsiveness to diuretics. The diuretic dose was adjusted by integrating the patient weight (as an indirect measure of fluid gain) with the self-reported degree of dyspnea, physical findings and capillary oxygen saturation. As needed, an additional diuretic (metolazone) was added to potentiate the effect. For ensuring minimal alterations of the measured subjects' posture and associated volume conductor geometry, all measurements were taken while in a sitting position, during tidal respiration. The electrode belt was attached to the patients' thorax on the plane of the fifth intercostal space in the midclavicular line (Figure 7).

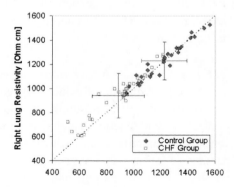

Figure 5. A scatter plot of right vs. left lung resistivity reconstruction values for control and CHF groups (Zlochiver et al. 2005, needs permission)

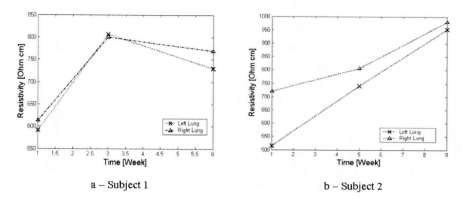

a – Subject 1   b – Subject 2

Figure 6. Left and right lung resistivity reconstruction values as a function of measurement time in weeks for (a) subject 1 and (b) subject 2 (Zlochiver et al. 2005, needs permission)

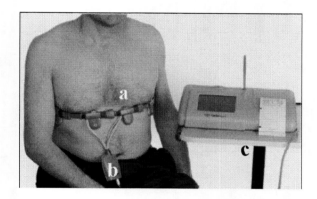

Figure 7. A typical measurement session. An eight-electrode thoracic belt (a) is attached to a sitting patient, and connected through an analogue driving and amplification unit (b) to a control/display unit (c). Freimark et al. 2007 (needs permission)

The electrode belt was removed between measurements. The urine output of the patients in the time interval between the two measurements was also measured for comparison.

The bio-impedance measurements before the intravenous diuretics treatment and following the resting period are shown in Figure 8 for all 13 patients. The upper, middle and lower graphs relate to the left-, right- and average-lung resistivity values. It can be seen that in all cases but one the post-treatment measurement indicated an increase in the resistivity value of both lungs (resistivity increase median value—8%, 25 percentile—4.75%, 75 percentile—14.25%), which corresponded to a dehydration of the lungs, as expected from the diuretics treatment. These changes cannot be attributed to measurement inconsistency, as we have already shown that the system reproducibility, both within and between tests, is better than 2%, in a 5 month monitoring period (see 3.2.1). A correlation graph between the absolute change in lung resistivity and the urine output is given in Figure 9, demonstrating a significant linear relationship with a correlation ratio of R = 0.73 (p = 0.004). A regression plot of the relative lung resistivity change (as a percentage) as a function of the urine output also demonstrated a significant linear relationship with a correlation ratio of R = 0.64 (p < 0.02).

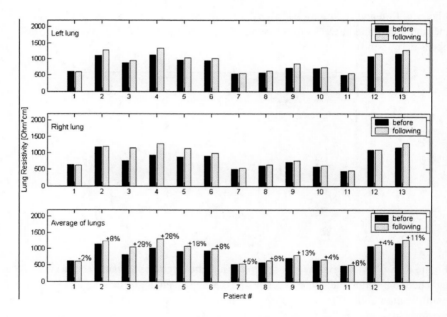

Figure 8. Left (up), right (middle) and average (bottom) lung resistivity measurements before (dark bars) and following (light bars) diuretics treatment. The change in the average lung resistivity as a percentage is noted (Freimark et al. 2007, needs permission).

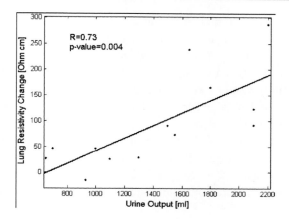

Figure 9. Correlation plot between average lung resistivity change and urine output (Freimark et al. 2007, needs permission).

3.2.4. Correlation between bio-impedance measurements and X-ray radiographs

To further support the validity of the bio-impedance measurements in monitoring CHF patients, a clinical study was conducted in which these new measurements were compared to standard X-ray radiograph scores. The study comprised of 14 patients (mean age 79±10 yr, n=9 females / 5 males) with clinical signs of pulmonary congestion of varying degrees, that were hospitalized in the departments of internal or geriatric medicine in Sheba Medical Center, Israel. The study was approved by a local ethics committee. Patients' condition was diagnosed by medical history, physical findings, chest radiography, electrocardiogram and echocardiography. None of the patients had history or clinical signs of chronic pulmonary disease (such as chronic obstructive pulmonary disease, pulmonary emphysema, tuberculosis or idiopathic pulmonary fibrosis). All patients with acute pulmonary infection and those carrying a cardiac pacemaker or other implantable devices were excluded from the study. Eight of the 14 patients had coronary artery disease (7 with old myocardial infarction, and 1 with coronary artery bypass grafting), 2 had obstructive cardiomyopathy, and the other four patients suffered from valvular heart diseases. All patients signed an informed consent. As before, measurements were performed while the patient was sitting, and had a short rest to ensure shallow tidal volume respiration with minimal movement of the thoracic cavity. The belt was attached around the chest on the plane of the fifth intercostals space in the mid-clavicular line. Each patient was studied at two time points resulting in a total of 28 measurements. An initial pre-furosemide measurement was taken as a reference measurement. A second measurement following the appropriate treatment to reduce pulmonary congestion was taken within 12 hours of furosemide dose. The mean of the reconstructed left and right lung resistivity values were stored for analysis. Standard upright chest x-ray radiographs were obtained in all patients at the reference time point and following treatment. The 28 radiographs were examined independently by a radiography expert blinded to the results of the clinical examination or the bio-impedance data. A semi-quantitative evaluation of radiographic appearance was determined by using a reading table, developed by Balbarini et al. (1991) and consisting of various radiographic findings indicative of pulmonary edema (table 2).

Table 2. Radiographic criteria (Balbarini et al. 1991) used to grade pulmonary interstitial edema.

X-Ray findings	Rating	Score
Hilar enlargement	0	0
	+	8
	++	10
	+++	12
Hilar density	0	0
	+	6
	++	12
Hilar blurring	0	0
	+	8
	++	10
Peribronchial cuffs	0	0
	+	10
Kerley lines	0	0
	+	10
Micronodules	0	0
	+	10
Widening of fissures	0	0
	+	8
Subpleural effusion	0	0
	+	6
Diffuse increase of opacity	0	0
	+	6
Extensive perihilar haze	0	0
	+	4

The mean lung bio-impedance measurements at the reference and post-treatment phases are summarized in table 3. Significant differences in the mean left and right lung resistivity values (a total of 28 measurements, two per patient, that include pre and post treatment values), were found between patients who were clinically diagnosed by the physician as suffering from high level pulmonary congestion and those diagnosed with a low level: 838±133 Ωcm (n=10 measurements) vs. 1002±164 Ωcm (n=18 measurements), respectively; p<0.01. Figure 10 shows representative examples of chest X-ray radiographs from the same patient before (left panel) and following (right panel) treatment. Significant changes in both radiographic scores and lung resistivity values were obtained. A significant difference was found in the bio-impedance measurements between the mean lung resistivity following pharmacological treatment and the reference value: 943±300 vs. 853±435 Ωcm (p-value<0.01, paired t-test). In contrast, the radiographic score did not exhibit significant difference between the two measurement phases – 23.4±22 vs. 25.4±25 (p-value>0.05, paired t-test). These results demonstrate the higher sensitivity of the bio-impedance approach in diagnosing pulmonary congestion than the standard radiographic score. In the next stage, we categorized the bio-impedance measurements that were taken at the reference phase (i.e. pre-treatment) and the measurements that were taken post-treatment according to the corresponding radiographic score. Two sub-groups were considered – measurements corresponding to a radiographic score lower than 20 ("light congestion") and those that correspond to higher radiographic scores ("severe congestion"). In the pre-treatment, reference phase, a significant difference was found between the means of the bio-impedance measurements between the two subgroups: 777±102 vs. 954±107 Ωcm for the severe and light congestion subgroups, respectively (p-value<0.01, unpaired t-test). On the other, no significant difference of means was found for the post-treatment measurements (887±183 vs. 999±174 Ωcm, for the severe and light congestion subgroups, respectively). The diagnostic value of the bio-impedance technique and its feasibility in differentiating congested and treated patients was thus demonstrated. The bio-impedance measurements were also capable of monitoring the degree of improvement in pulmonary congestion of individual patients. As seen in Figure 11, a significant correlation existed between the change in mean lung resistivity at the two time points (i.e. the reference measurement and following treatment) and the corresponding difference in the radiographic score (R=0.57, p<0.04). 5 out of 14 pharmacologically treated patients received a higher radiographic score with comparison to the reference

Table 3. Bio-impedance measurement and radiographic scores.

Patient #	Reference measurement		Post-treatment measurement	
	Mean lung resistivity [Ωcm]	Radiographic score	Mean lung resistivity [Ωcm]	Radiographic score
1	853	20	800	38
2	1083	0	1231	0
3	824	24	889	34
4	715	48	834	36
5	829	0	819	0
6	625	38	675	58
7	861	13	1200	38
8	1060	10	1061	44
9	910	68	1206	10
10	771	64	852	16
11	660	54	753	54
12	884	0	935	0
13	996	0	1089	0
14	871	16	859	0

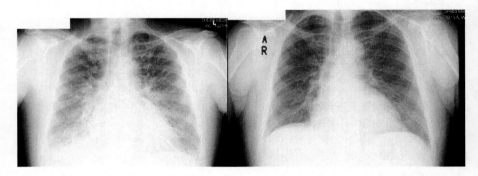

Figure 10. Representative chest X-ray radiographs. Left – a patient suffering from high degree of pulmonary congestion with a quantitative evaluation score of 68 and mean left and right lung resistivity values of 910 Ωcm. Right - The x-ray chest radiograph from the same patient following treatment (quantitative evaluation score of 10 and mean left and right lung resistivity values of 1206 Ωcm). Arad et al. 2009 (needs permission).

score (thus implying an improvement in congestion), while a much higher number of 10 out of 14 patients exhibited a clear improvement in their mean lung resistivity measurement (defined as a difference between measurements higher than 50 Ωcm. These results demonstrated again the higher sensitivity and specificity of the bio-impedance measurement with respect to the standard radiographic score.

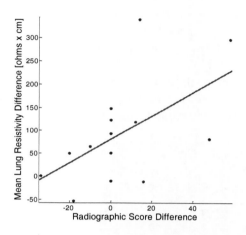

Figure 11. A correlation plot of the difference in mean left and right lung resistivity values between measurements versus the difference in radiographic score (n=14). Arad et al. 2009 (needs permission).

3.3. Monitoring CHF Patients at Home Via a Telemedicine Approach

An important advantage of the bio-impedance technique for monitoring CHF patients is the compactness, low-cost and user friendly realization of the commercial system. These features imply that CHF patients can be monitored at their home, without having to frequently visit the local clinic and, in many cases, without the need for a physician or nurse assistance. As a result, not only substantial hospitalization costs are saved, but also the quality of life of these patients can potentially improve significantly. In view of this potential, we have developed a telemedicine system that was based on a similar bio-impedance hybrid system as described above, that allows lung impedance measurements to be taken by the patient at the privacy and convenience of its home, and the online transmission of the taken measurements to a medical call center for analysis and professional diagnostics. The system (PulmoTrace@Home™, CardioInspect, Tel-Aviv University, Tel-Aviv, Israel) is composed of the following three main parts: (1) Two measurement units that contain 4 disposable electrodes mounted in pairs on a semi-flexible chest contraption, aimed to ensure that the electrodes will be attached at the same position in every measurement, (2) a portable unit that contains a controller that generates the measurement sequence, an analog unit which injects the current, performs voltage measurement, and measures the ECG signal, and two status LEDs to inform the patient about the measurement status, errors that might occur and the battery state. The unit is powered by a chargeable battery allowing for more than one hour of operation, and (3) a cradle that includes an internal modem for the transmission of the measured data, and a charger for the battery in the portable unit (Figure 12).

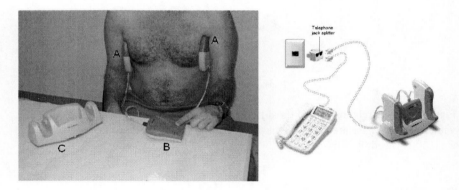

Figure 12. The telemedicine system. Left – measuring phase, right – schematics of the transmission phase. A – the two measurements units, B – the portable unit, C – the cradle. Radai et al. 2008 (needs permission).

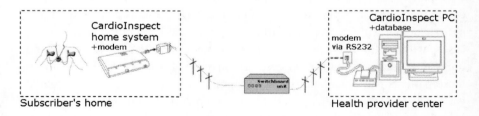

Figure 13. A schematic illustration of the telemedicine system (Radai et al. 2008, needs permission).

The self-measurement is done by first attaching the two measurement units to their right position on the patient's thorax, and pressing a button for starting the measurement. The hardware ensures a proper contact of the electrodes, and records 7 seconds of one-lead ECG, using a 12-bit resolution analog-to-digital converter (ADC) at a sampling-rate of 200Hz. Subsequently an impedance measurement is performed: two opposite (transthoracic) current injections are performed, each followed by a voltage measurement from the other two electrodes. The measured data is then transmitted via the physical telephone line connection, which is expected to be found at any patient home, into a Call-Center – at the health provider center (Figure 13). The Call-Center is composed of a personal computer containing a Microsoft-Access based database to maintain all personal information of the patients and the receiving data from the measurements. A Visual Basic.NET program is responsible of receiving the incoming data, adding it to the existing database, and handling the database. Once the measured data arrive at the Call-Center they are processed in offline mode to extract the following parameters: resistivity values of the left and right lungs from the impedance measurement, heart-rate, RR-interval, QT-interval and corrected QT-interval from the 7 seconds of the recorded one-lead ECG.

All incoming data is transmitted into a health provider center, which is responsible of collecting, saving and analyzing it. The Microsoft-Access based database contains two tables: one that stores personal details of the patients such as ID number, full name, admission date, birth-date, gender, height, weight at admission (as a reference value), chest circumference, address and other contact information. The second table contains the results of the examinations, and stores them in the following fields: date and hour of the examination, left and right lung resistivity values, RR-interval, QT-interval, and the file-name containing the ECG record. Figure 14 shows an example of surveillance after a healthy subject, which was recorded using the PulmoTrace@Home™ system along a period of about 6 weeks.

A preliminary clinical experiment was conducted on a small group of 5 healthy men, in order to demonstrate the feasibility of the presented telemedicine system, and its consistency in making resistivity measurements. Six resistivity measurements were taken for each subject, every 48 hours. Figure 15 shows the resulted resistivity values as were received at the Call-Center. As can be seen, the resistivity measurements are quiet consistent, as represented by the STD value of each subject, with a mean value of the STDs of 67 Ω cm.

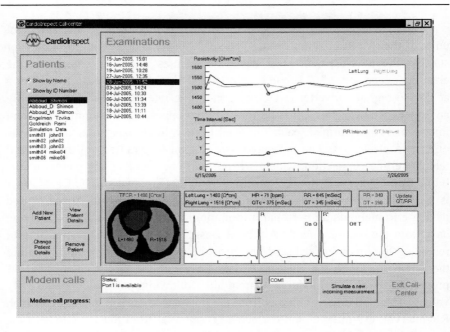

Figure 14. Surveillance after a healthy subject, as received via the telemedicine system (Radai et al. 2008, needs permission).

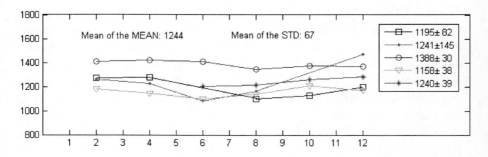

Figure 15. Measured resistivity values of five healthy males, taken by the telemedicine system. The measurements were taken six times, every 48 hours (Radai et al. 2008, needs permission).

Ten elderly patients (4 men, 6 women, age 76.1±11.7 years, from the Department of Geriatric Rehabilitation, Sheba Medical Center, Israel) suffering from Pulmonary Congestion were measured using the bio-impedance system. Patients' condition was diagnosed by medical history, physical findings, chest radiography, electrocardiogram and echocardiography. We have excluded all patients carrying a cardiac pacemaker or other implantable devices. Nine out of the 10 patients had coronary artery disease and one patient suffered from valvular heart disease. Their mean resistivity values were significantly lower than those of the healthy subjects - 887 ± 117 Ω cm vs. 1244 ± 87 Ω cm (p<0.01).

4. SUMMARY AND CONCLUSIONS

In this chapter, a portable stand-alone bio-impedance system for monitoring lung resistivity was designed and built, and its performances were evaluated on a healthy population as well as on CHF patients. An emphasis was placed for designing a light, user-friendly, self-operated and real-time system that would be easily fitted in both clinical and home environments. The bio-impedance technique, which was implemented in the present system, provides a safe and relatively cheap alternative to existing monitoring methods, and in the case of monitoring lung fluids, it overcomes much of their limitations. In addition, the compact size of the system and its usage simplicity suggest its suitability for both clinical and home environment application. As such, the currently burdensome necessity of many lung edema patients of being regularly monitored at the hospital may be avoided in the near future, which besides the improvement of life quality will save considerable hospitalization costs.

The hybrid bio-impedance approach, utilized in this study, combines the advantages of the two currently common approaches, i.e. the transthoracic impedance measurement and EIT, yet avoiding their characteristic limitations. As opposed to the transthoracic measurement, this approach offers specific left and right-lung resistivity values, while using only a small number of electrodes and fixed model geometry, thus avoiding the inherent EIT instability and ill-posedeness difficulties. The lung reconstruction algorithms that were implemented in the present system incorporated forward and inverse solvers. The forward solver was based on the finite volume method (FVM), which is conveniently suited for flow conservation problems such as in this case due to its integral, rather than differential, formulation. By directly solving the integral equations, the FVM is also appropriate for piecewise resistivity distributions, as exist in biological volume conductors. In many applications, this method requires less computational resources and CPU time than other numerical methods, e.g. the finite element or boundary methods (Lucquin and

Pironneau 1998). The inverse solver algorithm that was implemented was based on an iterative parametric Newton–Raphson scheme. This second order method usually provides better reconstruction quality than first-order, linear schemes, e.g. back-projection or simple inverse-matrix multiplication in terms of absolute resistivity values reconstruction. A major drawback of the iterative scheme originates from the long reconstruction times, especially when all pixels (or voxels in the three-dimensional case) in the volume conductor domain need to be reconstructed. In addition, a successful convergence usually requires regularization to compensate for the ill-conditioning of the Hessian matrix, needed to be inverted in the iterative procedure, which is related to the ill-posedeness of the inverse problem. The ill-conditioning makes the inverse-solver extremely sensitive to the accuracy of the knowledge of the boundary profile and the electrode positions. Since here we were only interested in monitoring lung resistivity, we had imposed a priori knowledge of the volume conductor geometry and resistivity properties, which were assumed constant for all subjects, and limited the optimization to only two parameters—the resistivity of the right and left lungs. By doing so, the reconstruction time and the inverse scheme stability were improved significantly, on the expense of geometrical model complexity, which was considered two-dimensional. This is naturally a simplification of the three-dimensional body, but still, appropriate for approximating three-dimensional cylindrical bodies such as the thoracic cavity. To adapt the two-dimensional forward problem solver calculations during the iterative reconstruction process to the physically measured electrode voltages, a calibration was required, in which a scaling factor was used to adapt the mean lung resistivity value of healthy subjects to the value reported in literature. In other works, direct calibrations are done to allow absolute imaging, e.g. by matching the calculated voltages of the forward solver to the measured EIT voltages, and by fitting the geometry model to the subjects' anthropometric parameters (Brown et al. 2002). Such an approach may be required for full reconstruction problems, where the accuracy of the geometrical model must be high. In the present approach, on the other hand, in which only the lungs' properties are directly reconstructed, a constant two-dimensional model was found sufficient, as an analysis of the correlation between the reconstructed mean resistivity values and various anthropometric parameters has shown independency. This implies that no further calibration or normalization of the measured quantities was needed. Moreover, this also implies that any significant change in the reconstructed values most probably indicate a pathological condition, which reflects in a lung resistivity variation. As the results show, the within-test and between-test reproducibility were both under 2%, again emphasizing that the exact knowledge of the geometry and electrode positions were no more such a crucial aspect as in other, full pixel reconstruction EIT systems. It was found that the mean and standard deviation of the left and right-lung reconstructed resistivity values were balanced, as expected for normal population, confirming the appropriateness of the suggested model and the reconstruction algorithm. In addition, the good reproducibility of the system did not come in expense for the dynamic range of the measured lung resistivity values. This was checked by monitoring the lung resistivity values of 11 healthy subjects during respiration. Mean lung resistivity changes of $50\pm12\%$ between tidal respiration and half inspirium and $72\pm12\%$ between tidal respiration and full inspirium were found. Another aspect concerns the medicinal treatment of CPE patients, which is intended to reduce the cardiac workload, enhance the myocardial contractility, and control of excessive retention of salt and water. The latter purpose is achieved by giving diuretic agents, however, over-treatment with diuretics must be avoided, since the resultant hypovolemia may reduce cardiac output, interfere with renal function and produce profound weakness and lethargy. Diuretics might also reduce the concentration of important ions in the blood circulation, causing phenomena such as hypokalemia. These symptoms are accompanied with ECG waveform changes, most prominently a prolongation of the QT interval (Isselbacher et al. 1994), and therefore measuring and tracking changes in the QT interval using signal processing techniques can give an indication to an overdose of the given diuretics. The present system has the capability to provide this additional diagnostic information from the ECG signal (e.g. QT and RR intervals), thus improving diagnostic value and consequently allowing a better adjustment of the medical treatment.

A significant separation of mean lung resistivity value between a control and a CHF group was found, showing the capability of the system to classify the patients. This separation probably resulted from the pathology condition of the CHF group, since as already noted, no dependence was found between the lung resistivity of the control group and their anthropometric parameters. Furthermore, additional external factors e.g. smoking or pulmonary disease at baseline did not bias the observed results, as no such conditions were dominant in the study group. It was found that while the left and right-lung reconstructed resistivity values were balanced for the control group, the right lung seemed to be associated with a higher resistivity than the left lung for the CHF group. Although this imbalance was not found to be significant ($p=0.23$), it is still an interesting finding, the physiological origins of which should be further studied. Unilateral pulmonary edema and pathological conditions such as unilateral pleural effusion are possible origins for the left-right lung resistivity asymmetry; however, these conditions were scarce among the CHF study group (only 6 out of 34 patients had pleural effusion), thus such a correlation could not be tracked. Another possible origin for the observed asymmetry would be an enlarged cardiac volume. Due to the low resistivity of the heart, such pathology can be interpreted by the parametric reconstruction algorithm used in the present system, in which the lungs' geometry was assumed constant, as a reduced left-lung resistivity. Indeed, the mean end-diastolic and end-systolic volumes in the group of CHF patients were 203ml and 129ml in respect, considerably larger than the normal values of 120ml and 50ml (Guyton 1991). The systems' capability for long-term monitoring edema severity was generally demonstrated on two CHF patients. The results, which showed a gradual decrease in the reconstructed lungs' resistivity, were correlated with both weight decrease and physician's diagnosis, suggesting the present system as an alternative system for CHF monitoring over long periods. Due to the limited scope of this monitoring phase, no conclusive comments are intended to be established at this point, although the preliminary outcome is encouraging and coherent with the expected theoretical trends.

The feasibility and validity of the bio-impedance measurements in monitoring CHF patients was also studied in conjunction with both urine output of patients undergoing diuretics treatment and with expert diagnosis using conventional X-ray radiographs. Regarding the former test, the clinical study that was conducted on CHF patients revealed a lung resistivity increase with a median value of 8% following intravenous diuretics treatment, indicating an improvement in their condition. In addition, a significant correlation between lung resistivity changes and urine output of $R = 0.73$ ($p = 0.004$) was demonstrated. These results were in accordance with those found for a group of healthy volunteers (Noble et al 2000), where an increase of 7.8% in right-lung impedance was found following fluid depletion and a correlation between lung impedance and urine output was demonstrated. Pulmonary edema in healthy subjects, created under experimental conditions or clinical situations (e.g. Tachyarrhythmia, extreme volume overload), produces a brisk diuretic response mediated by neurohumoral mechanisms: release of natriuretic peptide and decreased excretion of antidiuretic hormone. In heart failure patients these regulatory mechanisms are attenuated and even suppressed by other stimuli evoked by abnormal hemodynamics: low cardiac output, decreased renal perfusion, activated sympathetic and renin–angiotensin system and multiple medications affecting the renal and neurohumoral function. In heart failure excess fluid accumulates in blood vessels (i.e. venous congestion) tissue interstitium (i.e. edema involving the lungs, extremities, intestine, etc) and third spaces (pleural effusion or ascitis). The distribution of volume overload is highly variable and depends on type and chronicity of heart failure as well as nutritional status, liver and kidney function and local factors. During diuretic therapy fluid is mobilized first from the intravascular compartment, then from the interstitium and finally from body cavities. The water content of the lungs is only one factor related to urine output under diuretic therapy. However, since there is a gross correlation between the degree of lung congestion and general fluid overload in CHF, there should be a positive correlation between fluid loss and decrease in lung water content. A correlation of 0.73 (explaining more than 50% of experimental variance) is rather remarkable given the complex distribution of excess water in advanced heart failure. In one of our measurements, a negative resistivity change was recorded (see Figure 8, patient 1) for a patient with a urine output of ~900 ml. Such a negative change was most probably a result of a misconducted measurement, which may have occurred due to abrupt patient movement. The current results clearly demonstrate the feasibility of the hybrid bio-impedance system for long-term monitoring of CHF patients and its diagnostic value. As the system capability to separate between normal and CHF conditions was demonstrated, and its reproducibility was found to be better than 2%, the resistivity changes following diuretics treatment of up to 300 Ωcm, which are up to 25% of the reference lung resistivity values, were significant. The large inter-patient variability that was observed in the impedance changes was thus directly correlated to the urine output. Excess fluid, salt and caffeine and in particular hydration status could have influenced the urine output. However, because the patients were under a steady and restricted drinking and diet regimen, which included a hospital meal on the study day, these factors could not have been a major source of variability in this study.

With respect to the comparison of the bio-impedance diagnostic value to that of conventional X-ray radiographs, the bio-impedance system was successful in monitoring changes in patients' condition, exhibiting a significant correlation with the changes of the radiographic scores. In addition, the bio-impedance technique was found more sensitive to the congestion status of the patients, exhibiting a significantly higher lung resistivity value following the pharmacological treatment, while no significant corresponding radiographic score differences. Moreover, the bio-impedance technique successfully diagnosed an improvement of congestion level in 10 out of 14 patients, while the radiographic score indicated such an improvement in only 5 out of the 14 patients. These results further support the previous validation studies reported here.

In addition to monitoring lung resistivity as an indicator to pulmonary congestion and edema, we have previously demonstrated in a preliminary study the capability of the bio-impedance system to assess stroke volume, which is another important diagnostic indicator for CHF patients. In Zlochiver et al. (2006) we compared the performance of the PulmoTrace bio-impedance system with that of the BioZ impedance cardiography (by Cardiodynamics) and showed a correlation of r=0.86 (p-value=4x10^{-9}, N=28 subjects).

The telemedicine version of the system was developed in accordance with many previous studies showing that home telemedicine presents clear advantages to the well-being of CHF patients. Telemedicine companies recognize the importance of assessing the patient's edema level as a predictive indicator for re-hospitalization, and therefore all include in their devices either weight or subjective questionnaire as a measure to pulmonary edema (PE). Although weight can be easily measured by the user, it is a poor indicator to PE itself, as it might reflect many other pathologies or physiological processes that do not originate or relate to PE. Subjective questions to the patient are clearly not accurate enough and are highly dependent on psychological variable. In choosing the means of transporting the data from the patient's home to the medical center, several considerations were made, mainly abundance and simplicity of use. A simple modem seemed to provide the best answer. Aside from being reliable and cheap, it requires only a regular phone-line that can be found at any western home, in contrast to alternatives such as internet or cellular communication, which might not be found, especially among the elderly population. Moreover, a simple modem allowed for a very simple use - pressing a button placed on the portable unit, without the need of learning new skills such as operating a complicated cellular-phone, or facing the burdensome internet communication. Finally, a modem is also very suitable due to the small amount of data that is sent (~3kbyte) and thus the low transmission rates needed.

In conclusion, the results presented in this chapter are all consistent and suggest that by employing the bio-impedance and parametric EIT principles, a convenient, non-invasive, reproducible and safe monitoring of lung edema is feasible, which goes some way toward achieving the 'ideal' CHF monitoring device envisaged by Staub (1986). A system following individual chest impedance provides important additional information about lung water excess, which is relatively free of confounders complicating the currently used clinical measures.

REFERENCES

American Heart Association, Heart Disease and Stroke Statistics – 2005 Update. Available at *http://www.americanheart.org/downloadable/heart*

Arad M, Zlochiver S, Davidson T, Shovman O, Shoenfeld Y, Adunsky A and Abboud S 2009 Estimating pulmonary congestion in elderly patients using bio-impedance technique: correlation with clinical examination and X-ray results Med Eng Phys in-press

Balbarini A, Limbruno U, Bertoli D, Tartarini G, Baglini R, Mariotti R, Pistolesi M and Mariani M 1991 Evaluation of pulmonary vascular pressures in cardiac patients: the role of the chest roentgenogram J Thorac Imaging. 6 62-68

Bazett HC 1920 An analysis of the time-relations of electrocardiograms Heart 7 353

Brown BH, Barber DC and Seagar AD 1985 Applied potential tomography: possible clinical applications Clin Phys Physiol Meas 6 109–21

Brown B. Review of EIT systems available for medical use. In: Holder D, editor. Clinical and physiological applications of electrical impedance tomography. London, UK: UCL Press; 1993. p. 41–5.

Brown B H, Flewelling R, Griffiths H, Harris N D, Leathard A D, Lu L, Morice A H, Neufeld G R, Nopp P and Wang W 1996 EITS changes following oleic acid induced lung water Physiol. Meas. 17 A117–30

Brown BH, Primhak RA, Smallwood RH, Milnes P, Narracott AJ and Jackson MJ 2002 Neonatal lungs: maturational changes in lung resistivity spectra Med Biol Eng Comput 40 506–11

Campbell J H, Harris N D, Zhang F, Brown B H and Morice A H 1994a Clinical applications of electrical impedance tomography in the monitoring of changes in intrathoracic fluid volumes Physiol. Meas. 15 A217–22

Campbell J H, Harris N D, Zhang F, Morice A H and Brown B H 1994b Detection of changes in intrathoracic fluid in man using electrical impedance tomography Clin. Sci. 87 97–101

Chakko S, Woska D, Martinez H, de Marchena E, Futterman L, Kessler KM and Myerberg RJ 1991 Clinical, radiographic, and hemodynamic correlations in chronic congestive heart failure: conflicting results may lead to inappropriate care Am J Med. 90 353-359

Charach G, Rabinovich P, Grosskopf I andWeintraubM2001 Transthoracic monitoring of the impedance of the right lung in patients with cardiogenic pulmonary edema Crit. Care Med. 29 1137–44

Fein A, Grossman R F, Jones J G, Goodman P C andMurray J F 1979 Evaluation of transthoracic electrical impedance in the diagnosis of pulmonary edema Circulation 60 1156–60

Freimark D, Arad M, Sokolover R, Zlochiver S and Abboud S 2007 Monitoring lung fluid content in CHF patients under intravenous diuretics treatment using bio-impedance measurements Physiol Meas 28 S269-S277

Frerichs I, Hahn G, Schroder T and Hellige G 1998 Electrical impedance tomography in monitoring experimental lung injury Intens. Care Med. 24 829–36

Gabriel S, Lau RW and Gabriel C 1996 The dielectric properties of biological tissues", Parts I–III. Phys Med Biol 2231–93. Online database at: http://niremf.ifac.cnr.it/tissprop/ (October 2004).

Gehlbach BK and Geppert E 2004 The pulmonary manifestations of left heart failure Chest. 125 669-682

Grimnes S and Martinsen ØG. Bioimpedance and bioelectricity basics. San Diego, CA: Academic Press; 2000.

Guyton A C 1991 Textbook of Medical Physiology 8th edn (Philadelphia, PA: Saunders) pp 419–20

Harris ND, Suggett AJ, Barber DC and Brown BH 1987 Applications of applied potential tomography (APT) in respiratory medicine Clin Phys Physiol Meas 8(Suppl A) 155–65

Harris ND, Suggett AJ, Barber DC and Brown BH 1988 Applied potential tomography: a new technique for monitoring pulmonary function ClinPhys Physiol Meas 9(Suppl A) 79–85

Hayes CE, Case TA, Ailion DC, Morris AH, Cutillo A, Blackburn CW, Durney CH and Johnson SA 1982 Lung water quantitation by nuclear magnetic resonance imaging Science 216 1313-1315

Holder D, editor. Clinical and physiological applications of electrical impedance tomography. London, UK: UCL Press; 1993.

Hunt SA, Baker DW, Chin MH, *Cinquegrani MP, Feldman AM, Francis GS, Ganiats TG, Goldstein S, Gregoratos G, Jessup ML, Noble RJ, Packer M, Silver MA, Stevenson LW, Gibbons RJ, Antman EM, Alpert JS, Faxon, Fuster V, Gregoratos G, Jacobs AK, Hiratzka LF, Russell RO* and *Smith SC Jr* 2001 ACC/AHA Guidelines for the Evaluation and Management of Chronic Heart Failure in the Adult: Executive Summary A Report of the American College of Cardiology/American Heart Association Task Force on Practice Guidelines (Committee to Revise the 1995 Guidelines for the Evaluation and Management of Heart Failure): Developed in

Collaboration With the International Society for Heart and Lung Transplantation; Endorsed by the Heart Failure Society of America Circulation 104(24) 2996-3007

Isselbacher KJ, Braunwald E, Martin JB, Fauci AS,Wilson JD, Kasper DL, editors. Harrison's principles of internal medicine. 13th ed. New York, NY: McGraw-Hill; 1994.

Jongschaap HC, Wytch R, Hutchison JM and Kulkarni V 1994 Electrical impedance tomography: a review of current literature Eur J Radiol 18(3) 165–74

Kunst PW, Vonk Noordegraaf A, Straver B, Aart RA, Tesselaar CD, Postmus PE and de Vries 1998 Influences of lung parenchyma density and thoracic fluid on ventilatory EIT measurements Physiol Meas 19 27–34

Kunst P W A, Vonk-Noordegraaf A, Raaijmakers E, Bakker J, Groeneveld A B, Postmus P E and de Vries P M 1999 Electrical impedance tomography in the assessment of extravascular lung water in noncardiogenic acute respiratory failure Chest 116 1695–702

Liebman PR, Philips E, Weisel R, Ali J and Hechtman HB 1978 Diagnostic value of the portable chest x-ray technic in pulmonary edema Am J Surg. 135 604-606

Lucquin B, Pironneau O. Introduction to scientific computing. Chichester, NY: Wiley; 1998.

Morucci J P and Marsili P M 1996 Bioelectrical impedance techniques in medicine: Part III. Impedance imaging, second section: reconstruction algorithms Crit. Rev. Biomed. Eng. 24 599–654

Newell J C, Edic P M, Ren X, Larson-Wiseman J L and DanyleinkoMD 1996 Assessment of acute pulmonary edema in dogs by electrical impedance imaging IEEE Trans. Biomed. Eng. 43 133–8

Noble TJ, Morice AH, Channer KS, Milnes P, Harris ND and Brown BH 1999 Monitoring patients with left ventricular failure by electrical impedance tomography Eur J Heart Fail 1 379–84

Noble T J, Harris N D, Morice A H, Milnes P and Brown B H 2000 Diuretic induced change in lung water assessed by electrical impedance tomography Physiol. Meas. 21 155–63

Patroniti N, Bellari G, Massioni E, Manfio A, Marcora B and Pesenti A 2005 Measurement of pulmonary edema in patients with acute respiratory distress syndrome Crit Care Med. 33 2547-2554

Pomerantz M, Baumgartner R, Lauridson J and Eiseman B 1969 Transthoracic electrical impedance for the early detection of pulmonary edema Surgery 66 260–8

Radai MM, Abboud S and Rosenfeld M 1999 Evaluation of impedance technique for detecting breast carcinoma using a 2-D numerical model of the torso Ann NY Acad Sci 873 360–9

Radai MM, Abboud S and Rubinsky B 1999 Evaluation of the impedance technique for cryosurgery in a theoretical model of the head Cryobiology 38 51–9

Radai MM, Arad M, Zlochiver S, Krief H, Engelman T and Abboud S 2008 A novel telemedicine system for monitoring congestive heart failure patients Congestive Heart Fail 14 239-244

Saunders C E 1988 The use of transthoracic electrical bioimpedance in assessing thoracic fluid status in emergency department patients Am. J. Emerg. Med. 6 337–40

Schuller D, Mitchell J P, Calandrino F S and Schuster D P 1991 Fluid balance during pulmonary oedema Chest 100 1068–75

Staub N C 1986 Clinical use of lung water measurements Chest 90 588–94

Wang L and Patterson RP 1995 Multiple sources of the impedance cardiogram based on 3-D finite difference human thorax models IEEE Trans Biomed Eng 42 141–8

Yorkey TJ, Webster JG and Tompkins WJ 1987 Comparing reconstruction algorithms for electrical impedance tomography IEEE Trans Biomed Eng BME-34 843–52

Zellner J L, Spinale F G and Crawford F A 1990 Bioimpedance: a novelmethod for the determination of extravascular lung water J. Surg. Res. 48 454–59

Zlochiver S, Rosenfeld M and Abboud S 2003 Induced current electrical impedance tomography: a 2-D simulation of thoracic imaging IEEE Trans Med Imag 22 1550–60

Zlochiver S, Radai MM, Abboud S, Rosenfeld M, Dong X, Liu R, You FS, Xiang HY and Shi XT 2004 Induced current electrical impedance tomography system—experimental results and numerical simulations Physiol Meas 25 239–55

Zlochiver S, Radai MM, Barak-Shinar D, Ben-Gal T, Yaari V, Strasberg B and Abboud S 2005 Monitoring lung resistivity changes in congestive heart failure patients using the bioimpedance technique Congestive Heart Fail 11 289-293

Zlochiver S, Freimark D, Arad M, Adunsky A and Abboud S 2006 Parametric EIT for monitoring cardiac stroke volume Physiol Meas 27 S139-S146

Zlochiver S, Arad M, Radai MM, Barak-Shinar D, Krief H, Engelman T, Ben-Yehuda R, Adunsky A and Abboud S 2007 A portable bio-impedance system for monitoring lung resistivity Med Eng Phys 29 93-100

In: Congestive Heart Failure…   ISBN: 978-1-60876-677-2
Editors: J. E. García et al. pp. 37-60   © 2010 Nova Science Publishers, Inc.

Chapter 2

THE ASSOCIATION BETWEEN IMPLANTABLE CARDIOVERTER DEFIBRILLATOR SHOCKS AND HEART FAILURE: A REVIEW OF PATHOGENESIS AND MANAGEMENT

Alejandro Perez-Verdia, Sandra Rodriguez, Cihan Cevik and Kenneth Nugent

Texas Tech University Health Sciences Center, Department of Internal
Medicine, 3601 4th Street, Lubbock, TX 79430

ABSTRACT

The randomized trials with implantable cardioverter defibrillators
(ICDs) have demonstrated clear benefits for patients with
cardiomyopathy and systolic dysfunction. These trials have also provided
rich data sets from these patients and have identified management issues
which need more study. The MADIT II study demonstrated that ICDs
reduced all-cause mortality in patients with coronary disease and a low
ejection fraction. Appropriate shocks in this study predicted heart failure;
inappropriate shocks predicted an increase in all cause mortality. The
SCD-Heft study demonstrated that ICDs reduced all-cause mortality in
patients with ischemic and nonischemic cardiomyopathy. Patients
receiving both appropriate and inappropriate ICD shocks had an increase
in all-cause mortality compared to patients who did not receive shocks;

the most common cause of this mortality was heart failure. These two large studies demonstrate that ICD shocks are associated with heart failure progression. This may represent the natural history of these diseases, or it may represent the effect of shocks on myocardial function and/or interactions among shocks, the sympathetic nervous system, and psychiatric disorders associated with ICD use. Management issues include a careful selection of patients for ICD implantation. Other than the COMPANION study, randomized trials in patients with nonischemic cardiomyopathy do not demonstrate much benefit for those patients if they are on optimal medical therapy. ICDs need careful programming to limit the number of shocks and/or the energy required per shock. Medical management is crucial and should include beta-blockers and angiotensin converting enzyme inhibitors. The benefits with amiodarone therapy remain unclear in these patients. Physicians need to pay close attention to psychiatric symptoms with counseling, medication, and possible referral to psychiatrists. Cardiologists should use a standardized protocol to thoroughly review both the ICD device and medical care when these patients have shocks. More studies are needed on the importance of the New York Heart Association (NYHA) functional classification, psychiatric syndromes, and anti-arrhythmic medication use in these patients to limit complications and increase survival.

The Multicenter Automatic Defibrillator Implantation Trial (MADIT) published in 1996 demonstrated that implanted defibrillators (ICDs) improved survival in patients with ischemic cardiomyopathy when used as primary prevention [1]. The MADIT II and the Sudden Cardiac Death in Heart Failure Trial (SCD-HeFT) extended the indications for the use of ICDs, and current guidelines recommend ICD therapy for both primary and secondary prevention of sudden cardiac death as a Class I indication [2-4]. These trials have provided rich data sets from these patients with cardiomyopathy, have helped clarify the causes of mortality, and have identified management issues which need more study. The larger trials also demonstrate that ICD shocks have unintended effects on the natural history of heart failure, and we review these issues in this commentary.

1. MADIT II AND SCD-HEFT: TWO MAJOR RANDOMIZED CONTROLLED TRIALS OF IMPLANTABLE CARDIOVERTER-DEFIBRILLATOR THERAPY

The MADIT II compared ICD therapy with conventional medical therapy as primary prevention in 1352 patients with a left ventricular ejection fraction less than 30% and a history of previous myocardial infarction [2]. After an average of 20 months of follow-up, the mortality rates were 14.2% in the ICD group and 19.8% in the conventional medical therapy group (p=0.016). This represented a 31% reduction in the relative risk of mortality. There was an absolute reduction in the risk of all cause mortality of 5.6% at the end of the trial, and the number of patients needed to treat with an implanted ICD to prevent one death over two years was 18. This benefit was seen across all subgroups of NYHA functional class and QRS duration and persisted after adjustment for other covariates (hypertension, diabetes, atrial fibrillation, left bundle branch block, kidney functions, gender, age, and type of device). The benefit of ICD therapy did not become evident until the ninth month after implantation. Patients who met MADIT II criteria became eligible for ICD implantation per guidelines following the publication of this trial, and it was approved by Medicare as a reimbursable indication for ICD therapy.

The SCD-HeFT results confirmed the MADIT II results on the use of prophylactic ICDs in ischemic cardiomyopathy and extended the indications to patients with nonischemic cardiomyopathy [3]. The SCD-HeFT trial included 2521 patients with both ischemic and nonischemic cardiomyopathies. The mean follow up was longer at 45.5 months, and the mean LVEF was 25% for the overall study population (24% for the ICD group). In this trial there was an absolute risk reduction for overall mortality of 7.2% at five years (relative risk reduction of 23%). In contrast to the MADIT II trial, the overall benefit was lower and was limited to NYHA class II patients (70% of the study population) who had an absolute risk reduction of 11.9% and a relative risk reduction of 46%. Subgroup analyses did not identify any benefit for the NYHA class III patients (hazard ratio ICD vs. placebo, 1.16, 97.5% CI, 0.84-1.61, p=0.3). When the data were analyzed by etiology of heart failure, the risk reduction in the nonischemic group was marginal (p=0.06). Tung and coworkers suggested that the six interim analyses of the SCD-HeFT data should require a P value less than 0.025 for significance which then makes the risk reduction in the nonischemic cardiomyopathy patients even less

Clinical Trials

Acronym	Title	Publication Date
ATLAS	Assessment of Treatment With Lisinopril and Survival	1999
CAST	Cardiac Arrhythmia Suppression Trial	1989
CAST II	Cardiac Arrhythmia Suppression Trial II: Effect of the antiarrhythmic agent moricizine on survival after myocardial infarction	1992
CHARM	Candesartan in Heart Failure Assessment of Reduction in Mortality and Morbidity Alternative Trial	2003
CIBIS-II	The Cardiac Insufficiency Bisoprolol Study	1999
COMET	Carvedilol or Metoprolol European Trial	2003
COMPANION	Comparison of Medical Therapy, Pacing, and Defibrillation in Heart Failure	2004
CONSENSUS	Cooperative North Scandinavian Enalapril Survival Study	1987
COPERNICUS	The Carvedilol Prospective Randomized Cumulative Survival Study	2001
DEFINITE	Defibrillators in Non-Ischemic Cardiomyopathy Treatment Evaluation	2004
FEST	Fosinopril Efficacy Safety Trial	1995
IMPACT-HF	Initiation Management Predischarge: Process for Assessment of Carvedilol Therapy in Heart Failure	2004
MADIT I	Multicenter Automatic Defibrillator Implantation Trial	1996
MADIT II	Multicenter Automatic Defibrillator Implantation Trial II	2002
MERIT-HF	Metoprolol CR/XL Randomized Intervention Trial in Congestive Heart Failure	1999
Pain FREE Rx II	Pacing Fast Ventricular Tachycardia Reduces Shock Therapies	2004
PREPARE	Primary Prevention Parameters Evaluation Study	2008
RALES	Randomized Aldactone Evaluation Study Investigators	1999
SCD-HeFT	The Sudden Cardiac Death in Heart Failure Trial	2005
SOLVD	Studies of Left Ventricular Dysfunction	1991
STRETCH	Symptom, Tolerability, Response to Exercise Trial of Candesartan Cilexetil in Heart Failure	1999
SWORD	Survival With Oral d-Sotalol	1996
TOVA	Triggers of Ventricular Arrhythmias	2004
Val-HeFT	Valsartan Benefits Left Ventricular Structure and Function in Heart Failure Study	2001

significant [5]. This finding is consistent with other studies, such as the DEFINITE trial, that have exclusively studied the use of ICDs as primary prevention in nonischemic cardiomyopathy patients and have demonstrated a non-statistically significant reduction in mortality [6]. The patients treated with amiodarone did not benefit in the primary prevention of sudden cardiac death. Overall, the number needed to treat was 13 in SCD-HeFT, six in MADIT II, and two in MADIT at 5 years. The use of beta blockers and angiotensin converting enzyme (ACE) inhibitors/angiotensin receptor blocker (ARB) was higher in the SCD-HeFT study than in the MADIT II, and this could potentially explain the smaller reduction in death in the former.

2. PATHOGENESIS OF HEART FAILURE IN PATIENTS WITH ICD SHOCKS

The Effect of Shock: Appropriate and Inappropriate Shocks

ICDs can sense supraventricular rhythm disturbances as lethal ventricular arrhythmia and may deliver shocks inappropriately. Almost one-third of the shocks (184 of 590) delivered to the 719 MADIT II participants were classified as inappropriate. At least one inappropriate shock occurred in 11.5% of the patients with ICDs, and fifty-six patients (7.8%) had only inappropriate shock(s) [7]. The most common reason for inappropriate shocks was atrial fibrillation/flutter (44%) followed by supraventricular tachycardia (36%) and abnormal sensing (19%). Patients who received inappropriate shocks had a higher mortality (hazard ratio: 2.29, 95% confidence interval 1.11-4.71) than those who did not have inappropriate shocks. Hospitalization from heart failure was also higher in the ICD arm of MADIT II population (19.9% versus 14.9% over 20 months). This results in a number needed to harm of 20 (one excess hospitalization per 20 patients treated), suggesting that ICD therapy converts sudden death risk to a subsequent hospitalization for heart failure risk.

Poole and coworkers evaluated the long term (almost 4 years follow-up) prognostic significance of ICD shocks in SCD-HeFT participants. They demonstrated that patients with an ICD implanted for primary prevention have an increased mortality rate if they received appropriate and/or inappropriate ICD shocks [8]. In this study appropriate and inappropriate shocks were associated with a five-fold and two-fold increased risk of death, respectively. This risk increased by a factor of 11 in patients who received both shock types when compared to patients who received no shocks. Like the MADIT II results, the most common cause of increased mortality was worsening heart failure in the SCD-HeFT study (42.9%). Ventricular tachycardia/ventricular fibrillation, stroke, and acute coronary syndromes also cause death in these patients. Although the mortality benefit with ICDs occurs through the prevention of arrhythmic sudden cardiac death, these devices appeared to increase nonarrhythmic deaths in both trials.

The newer ICDs have more advanced sensing properties and can deliver more appropriate energy than the older models. However, regardless of the shock energy, ICDs still cause direct myocardial injury, contraction band necrosis, fibrosis, and possibly persistent inflammation [9]. Serum cardiac troponin I elevations (3.8 ± 4.3 ng/mL) occur in 43% of patients independent of any concurrent acute coronary syndrome after spontaneous ICD shocks [10]. Several episodes of ventricular fibrillation may be induced and terminated to test the correct sensing and defibrillation properties of the device during implantation. Therefore, 14% of patients have myocardial cell damage during the implantation of ICDs [11]. However, this practice has been changed significantly, since most clinicians currently induce ventricular fibrillation only once or twice during ICD implantation. On the other hand, the data regarding the number of shocks and troponin rise are also conflicting, and Hurst's study did not show any association between troponin rise and number of shocks in a multivariate analysis [11]. Studies in patients undergoing defibrillator implantation demonstrated that shocks higher than 9 joules reduce cardiac index by 10-15%, and this detrimental effect is proportional to the shock strength [12]. In addition to the myocardial damage from the shock itself, endocardial leads may cause foreign body reaction and enhance myocardial fibrosis. Increased fibrosis can increase defibrillation thresholds, and higher energy defibrillations will be required during subsequent arrhythmic events. These fibrotic areas may also lead to the development of new arrythmogenic reentry circuits. Although the pathological changes in the myocardium affect less than 2% of the total myocardial mass, these changes potentially contribute to more ventricular impairment since most of these patients already have severe left ventricular systolic dysfunction initially [9].

ICD Shocks and the Activation of Sympathetic Nervous System

Although the natural progression of heart failure will inevitably result in an increase in the number of appropriate and inappropriate shocks, activation of the autonomic nervous system during shocks also contributes to the increased mortality in these patients. Both external and internal defibrillation shocks activate the systemic sympathetic nervous system and increase overall sympathetic tone. Bode and coworkers investigated the effect of countershocks on cardiac and circulating catecholamines [13]. In this study, systemic adrenaline levels increased threefold following an ICD shock (10-34 joules, 30 patients). This dramatic increase was even more significant in patients after external defibrillation shocks. Moreover, comparison of arterial noradrenaline levels and coronary sinus noradrenaline levels demonstrated that cardiac noradrenaline uptake was significantly increased. This finding presumably reflects enhanced myocardial uptake of catecholamines following an ICD shock. Furthermore, these increased levels of systemic catecholamines persist for at least 10 minutes following the shock [14]. Catecholamines could cause direct myocardial cell damage through activation of calcium channels producing calcium overload and myocardial dysfunction, through acute oxidative stress, or through the induction of an acute inflammatory process. Persistently elevated plasma catecholamine levels could increase ventricular excitability, decrease the threshold for ventricular arrhythmias, and lead to more ICD shocks.

The Activation of Sympathetic Nervous System and the Psychiatric Consequences: Impact on Heart Failure Progression

Epidemiology. ICD shocks cause severe pain. Patients who have received ICD shocks after its implantation develop more anxiety, distress, and depression than those who have not had shocks [15]. The acute distress following an ICD shock may even result in posttraumatic stress disorder [16]. These patients feel sicker and closer to death regardless of their overall clinical condition. One third of the patients with ICDs have psychiatric disorders [17]. Mark and coworkers reported that patients have decreased quality of life, including emotional dysfunction, during the month following an ICD shock [18]. Similarly, the randomized, controlled Coronary Artery Bypass patch trial demonstrated that quality of life outcomes in ICD patients were worse than the outcomes in the patients without ICD [19]. The patients with ICD shocks had decreased physical and emotional role functioning and had lower levels of psychological well-being during the six months after their ICD placement. Frequent shocks, age less than 50, and female gender were risk factors for poor adjustment in ICD recipients in a national survey [17]. One possible explanation for these finding is that the shocks may remind the patients that they are ill and were near death during the recent ICD firing. It is not surprising that these psychiatric consequences can lead to unfortunate complications, including the possibility of suicide.

Explanation. Psychiatric disorders, including depression and anxiety, influence ischemic heart failure. Patients with chronic anxiety and depression have an activated hypothalamus-hypophysis-adrenal axis, increased sympathetic activity, and decreased vagal tone. Chronic sympathetic stimulation could directly affect the myocardium and increase cardiac dysfunction. Most patients with heart failure have a history of myocardial infarction as the etiology of their heart failure. Post myocardial infarction depression increases morbidity and mortality in patients with recent MI [20]. Furthermore, patients with ischemic heart disease and depression or anxiety are more likely to develop malignant ventricular arrhythmias. This association may be mediated by changes in the sympathetic nervous system, in vascular inflammation, and/or in platelet reactivity [21]. Panic disorder and agoraphobia are frequent side effects associated with ICD treatment [22]. Although its efficacy is limited in the treatment of panic disorder as a monotherapy, beta blocker therapy would be useful in these patients. The incidence of anxiety disorder was 6.9% even in patients who did not experience any shocks after ICD implantation (versus 21% in patients who had ICD shock). In this study new onset anxiety disorder developed in 16.7% of patients after ICD implantation. Other studies have also reported clinically diagnosable anxiety in 13-38% patients following ICD implantation, and, regardless of the baseline psychological status, 24-87% of ICD recipients will have more anxiety related symptoms after ICD implantation [17]. This, in turn, will increase the number of appropriate ICD shocks since the Triggers of Ventricular Arrhythmias (TOVA) study demonstrated that more severe symptoms of depression predicted ventricular arrhythmias and, accordingly, appropriate ICD shocks [23].

Anxiety and panic attacks have acute episodic presentations and have the potential to initiate cardiac syndromes. In general, these attacks are more common in women with a history of cardiovascular disease, chest pain, and/or depression and are associated with negative life events during the past year. Epinephrine is released from the heart at rest and during spontaneous attacks in patients with panic disorder [24]. Radiotracer studies using epinephrine and norepinephrine with collection of samples from the coronary sinus have demonstrated that patients with panic disorder have reduced extraction of norepinephrine and epinephrine during transit through the heart [25]. This has been attributed to impairment in the norepinephrine transporter which limits catecholamine effects on the heart by uptake. This abnormality has the potential to increase cardiac responses to catecholamine surges during panic attacks and other stressful events. In addition, changes in catecholamine kinetics could have regional effects independent of high circulating levels. Finally, studies in patients with panic attacks have demonstrated that induced panic attacks cause myocardial perfusion defects in patients with known coronary disease [26]. Severe stress with hyperadrenergic states can cause acute cardiac dysfunction in patients with normal coronary arteries (e.g., stress cardiomyopathy) and in patients with coronary artery disease. These studies suggest an important interaction among psychiatric disorders, stress-induced sympathetic states, and the worsening of heart failure after ICD implantation. This analysis has been presented in more detail in an earlier publication [27].

MANAGEMENT

Patients qualifying for ICD placement have advanced cardiac disease, and medical management is essential for good outcomes. We consider the core elements of patient management in this section.

Patient Selection

The current ACC/AHA guidelines for the implantation of ICDs clearly state that all patients who are to receive devices for the primary prevention of sudden death must be on optimal medical therapy and have a reasonable quality of life with a life expectancy of greater than one year [4]. The recommendations for implanting ICDs for primary prevention include:

(i) Patients with an ischemic cardiomyopathy with a prior myocardial infarction at least 40 days before implantation, with an EF of ≤35%, and NYHA functional class II-III or class I if the EF is ≤30%.

(ii) Patients with a non-ischemic cardiomyopathy with an EF of <35%.

(iii) Patients with an EF ≤40% due to prior myocardial infarction and non-sustained ventricular tachycardia who have inducible sustained VT or VF during an electrophysiological study.

The recommendations for secondary prevention include:

(i) Survivors of a sudden cardiac arrest due to VT/VF not due to a completely reversible cause.

(ii) Patients with structural heart disease and sustained VT whether hemodynamically stable or unstable.
(iii) Patients with syncope of unclear etiology with inducible sustained VT/VF during an electrophysiological study.

Except for the COMPANION trial, randomized controlled trials, including the SCD-HeFT trial, of patients with nonischemic dilated cardiomyopathy have not demonstrated that ICDs reduce all cause mortality [28, 29]. However, a meta-analysis of these trials did demonstrate that there is a reduction in all cause mortality with a relative risk for mortality of 0.69 (95% confidence in 0.55 − 0.87) [30]. This result remained statistically significant after the COMPANION trial was removed with a relative risk of 0.74 (95% CI − 0.58-0.96). Consequently, ICDs may provide less benefit in this patient population because their prognosis is relatively good with optimal medical therapy [29]. For example, the DEFINITE trial reported an annual mortality rate of 7 % in patients with nonischemic dilated cardiomyopathy treated with beta-blockers (85%) and ACE- inhibitors (86%) [6].

Optimal Medical Management of Heart Failure

The treatment of heart failure requires a multidisciplinary approach ranging from dietary recommendations to transplant evaluation. The current guidelines emphasize the importance of optimization of the medical therapy, weight control, regular follow-ups, and improving awareness of the clinical situation by patients and their family members. Optimal heart failure management requires the patients' understanding of worsening symptoms and their compliance with the adequate use of medications. First, good control of risk factors, such as hypertension, dyslipidemia, and diabetes mellitus, is crucial. Second, the ventricular rate needs to be optimized in patients with supraventricular arrhythmias. Third, smoking and alcohol consumption should be avoided. Finally, thyroid disorders or other endocrinopathies need to be treated, and the use of cardiotoxic medications such as cancer chemotherapy drugs needs to be reviewed at each follow-up.

In the current ACC/AHA guidelines, ACEIs, beta-blockers, diuretics, and salt restriction are class I recommendations for patients with heart failure [31]. ARBs can be used as alternative for ACE-inhibitor therapy if needed. Nonsteroidal anti-inflammatory drugs should be avoided. Maximal exercise testing should guide the exercise program and exercise training. Aldosterone antagonists can be added if the serum creatinine level is 2.5 mg/dl or less in men (2.0 or less in women), and the serum potassium is 5.0 mEq/L or less in patients with persistent symptoms. The addition of hydralazine/nitrates may be beneficial in African-American patients.

The ACEIs are the core drugs of heart failure treatment since they have improved morbidity and mortality in multiple trials. The Captopril-Digoxin Multicenter Research Group reported a significantly improved exercise time (mean increase 82 seconds vs. 35 seconds) and an improved NYHA class (41% vs. 22%) in patients who were treated with captopril instead of placebo [32]. In this study, the patients treated with digoxin did not achieve this level of improvement. This study was a landmark study with ACE inhibitor therapy in heart failure and caused a switch from digoxin to ACE inhibitors in these patients. The SOLVD study (1991) compared enalapril with placebo in patients with symptomatic congestive heart failure [33]. The mean duration of follow up was 41 months. This study demonstrated that addition of enalapril to the conventional treatment of patients with ejection fraction of less than 35% significantly improved clinical status and survival over placebo (reduction in risk, 16%; 95% confidence interval, 5% to 26%; P = 0.0036). The post hoc analysis of SOLVD revealed that NNT to prevent one death based on SOLVD results is 30 patient-years of drug intake. [34] Therefore, ACE inhibitors are recommended for all patients with heart failure due to left ventricle systolic dysfunction unless contraindicated.

ARBs are alternative drugs for patients who cannot tolerate ACEIs and have benefits similar to ACEIs in the clinical trials. The CHARM trial randomized 7601 people to either placebo or candesartan and followed them for a median duration of 37 months. [35] The overall mortality was 23% with candesartan and 25% with placebo. Candesartan significantly reduced covariate adjusted all-cause mortality (0.90 [0.82-0.99], p=0.032) and cardiovascular deaths (0.87 [0.78-0.96], p=0.006) compared to placebo. The Val-HeFT trial randomized 5010 patients to either valsartan or placebo [36]. Valsartan reduced the combined end-point of morbidity and mortality compared to placebo (relative risk, 0.87; 97.5 percent confidence interval, 0.77 to 0.97; P=0.009). This result can be summarized as treatment of 1000 patients for 2 years with valsartan would prevent 46 hospitalizations for worsening heart failure. The number needed to treat to prevent one event was 22.

Aldosterone antagonists have potential benefits in patients with either mild or advanced heart failure by blocking the effects of residual aldosterone since ACEIs fail to completely suppress this mineralocorticoid hormone. The addition of spironolactone to the standard therapy reduces the relative risk for death secondary to heart failure by 30% and the risk for hospitalization by 35% when compared to standard medical therapy in patients with Class III or IV heart failure. (RALES study, number needed to treat: 9) [37].

Beta-blockers such as bisoprolol, carvedilol, and metoprolol are strongly recommended for heart failure therapy. The COPERNICUS Trial randomly assigned 2289 patients with severe heart failure to either placebo or carvedilol for an average of 10 months (stopped prematurely) [38]. Carvedilol reduced the combined risk of death or hospitalization for a cardiovascular reason by 27% (P=0.00002) and the combined risk of death or hospitalization for heart failure by 31% (P=0.000004) compared to placebo. All cause mortality was reduced from 16% in the placebo arm to 11% in the carvedilol treatment arm (NNT 13, p<0.001). The MERIT-HF trial randomized 3991 patients with EF<40% to metoprolol CR/XL or placebo with a mean follow-up of one year (stopped prematurely) [39]. Metoprolol decreased all cause mortality at one year compared to placebo (7% vs. 10%, p<0.05, NNT of 29). Long term treatment with beta-blockers can reduce the risk of death and hospitalization and have additional beneficial effects when combined with ACE inhibitors.

Diuretics are useful in patients with heart failure and should be given to every patient who has a history or evidence of fluid retention. Diuretics produce symptomatic benefit more rapidly than any other drug for heart failure, reduce the risk of death and worsening heart failure, and improve exercise capacity [31].

Post hoc analysis of data from previous trials suggests that black or African descent patients have a good response to the combination of isosorbide dinitrate and hydralazine [31]. Adult black patients with EF of less than 35% (or less than 45% with an increased left ventricular internal end-diastolic diameter) have a significantly lower risk of death from any cause, a lower likelihood of first hospitalization for heart failure, and a greater improvement in quality of life scores. Hydralazine and nitrate combination can be used in any patient who cannot tolerate therapy with ACE inhibitor or ARB or who have renal insufficiency.

Device Programming

Understanding the profound adverse emotional impact and the potentially deleterious effects on myocardial function of implantable defibrillator shocks has led to different approaches to device programming to reduce the number of appropriate (but perhaps unnecessary) and inappropriate shocks. In both the

MADIT II and the SCD-HeFT trials approximately 30% of shocks were considered inappropriate, frequently due to supraventricular tachycardias erroneously classified as ventricular in origin by the devices. Several programmable features help reduce the risk of inappropriate shocks. These features vary among the different manufacturers, but all are effective to some degree. Antitachycardia pacing (ATP) is safe and effective in terminating the vast majority of slow ventricular tachycardias (<188 bpm) and many fast tachycardias (≥188 bpm). The Pain FREE Rx II Trial compared the use of ATP for tachycardias with rates between 188-250 bpm with shock as first line therapy [40]. This approach proved effective at terminating >70% of the tachycardias without an associated increased risk of syncope or acceleration to a faster tachycardia or ventricular fibrillation. Now most physicians programming these devices have adopted the use of ATP. However, this mode of therapy had not been used for the very fast tachycardias for fear of delaying treatment, and these rhythms had traditionally been treated with shocks first. The EnTrust clinical study investigators introduced the use of ATP while the device is charging the capacitors for delivery of a shock in the ventricular fibrillation zone [41]. This feature allowed the use of a single attempt at ATP without delaying the delivery of shock if the ATP failed to terminate the arrhythmia. ATP was successful in 69% of cases; it was more effective with monomorphic rhythms (likely VT) terminating 77% of them than polymorphic rhythms (likely VF) terminating 44%. This trial demonstrated the safety and efficacy of ATP even in patients with probable ventricular fibrillation episodes. This feature is available in newer devices. The mechanism for most ventricular tachycardias is a reentry circuit that self perpetuates. In general terms, ATP works by confronting the depolarizing wave front of the reentry circuit with a depolarizing front created by the pacing of the device which penetrates the tachycardia circuit and extinguishes it.

Another method for avoiding shocks is to avoid treating rhythms that are not sustained tachycardias. However, this approach had not been used for fear of allowing the patients to remain for long periods of time in a potentially dangerous rhythm. Until recently most devices had been programmed to allow only a certain number of beats ("number of intervals to detect") of the tachycardia in the programmed rate before the device delivered therapy. Physicians usually programmed this number at 18/24 and in some cases at 12/18. However, the PREPARE trial demonstrated that by prolonging these intervals to 30/40 there was a significant reduction in shocks (9% in study group vs. 17% in control group) without compromising safety [42]. The PREPARE trial, however, used patients from previous studies as its control group; hence it was not a head to head comparison. The ADVANCE III study is an ongoing trial in which is randomly and prospectively comparing the two strategies to determine the efficacy and safety of this more aggressive approach at programming ICDs [43].

Anti-Arrhythmic Medications, Including Amiodarone

Patients with heart failure are at risk for the development of tachyarrhythmias that have a high risk of sudden death; episodes of nonsustained ventricular tachycardia (VT), sustained VT, and supraventricular tachycardias can also cause progressive heart failure and increase mortality.

Standard heart failure therapy, as discussed in this commentary, decreases mortality. Beta-blockers which are classified as antiarrhythmic drugs in both the Vaughan- Williams and Sicilian Gambit systems reduce sudden death and all-cause mortality in both post infarction patients and patients with heart failure regardless of cause [44, 45]. However, other antiarrhythmic drugs have not improved survival and have increased mortality in some trials due to their proarrhythmic effects. The CAST study compared flecainide and encainide to placebo in patients post myocardial infarction to test the hypothesis that suppressing ventricular premature complexes improved mortality. However, there was increased relative risk (3.6x) of death in patients in the treatment group [46]. In the CAST II morizicine was used in a population with EF<40% to target a population with greater risk of arrhythmic mortality. This study was also prematurely terminated due to excess mortality in the treatment group [47]. The SWORD trial had a similar hypothesis but used d-sotalol, a pure potassium channel blocker, in post-myocardial infarction patients with depressed LVEF. It was also stopped early due to a significant increase in mortality in the treatment arm [48, 49]. The use of amiodarone in patients with CHF remains controversial. Some small studies and one meta-analysis have suggested a small survival benefit over placebo [50-52]. However, the SCD-HeFT showed no significant benefit compared to placebo and a worse outcome in the NYHA class III patients. Therefore, the routine use of antiarrhythmic drugs in the heart failure population as a primary prevention strategy is not recommended.

Patients with heart failure who receive implantable defibrillators are at risk for appropriate and inappropriate shocks. As discussed earlier, ICD shocks are associated with psychological distress, myocardial injury, and progression of heart failure. The question then arises: should we use antiarrhythmic drugs in those patients who have been implanted with an ICD to reduce their risk of shocks? The current guidelines do not advocate such an approach. Antiarrhythmic drugs have proarrhythmic side-effects and, hence, may increase the risk of ICD shocks; these drugs frequently have other important side-effects. The OPTIC trial compared the use of amiodarone and a beta-blocker, or sotalol alone, or beta-blocker alone in patients with depressed LV function who underwent ICD placement and who had sustained spontaneous or inducible VT/VF. In this particular trial amiodarone and beta-blocker were superior to beta-blocker alone in reducing the number of shocks (appropriate and inappropriate). Not surprisingly, this arm was associated with a statistically significant increase in adverse effects associated with amiodarone. The sotalol arm revealed a trend towards a reduction of shocks, but this did not reach statistical significance. There were no reported episodes of torsade de pointes with sotalol [53]. In a similar study by Pacifico and others sotalol significantly reduced shocks (appropriate and inappropriate) and overall death in a secondary prevention population with ICDs [54].

Currently antiarrhythmic drugs in the ICD population are reserved for suppression of atrial arrhythmias leading to progression of heart failure or inappropriate shocks and for patients who have repeated shocks from VT/VF storm. An ablative approach is also recommended for patients having recurrent inappropriate shocks secondary to supraventricular arrhythmias and for some patients with VT/VF storm to eliminate or reduce the arrhythmia burden.

Management of Psychiatric Symptoms and Syndromes

Anxiety, depression, and panic disorder are relatively common in the general population in the United States. These disorders are even more common in patients with chronic heart disease, especially if the patient cohort is identified during hospitalization. O'Connor and co-workers used the Beck depression inventory (BDI) to identify patients with depression during hospitalization for congestive heart failure [55]. Approximately 30% of these patients had a BDI score of greater than 10. Fifty-three percent of these patients died during a two and one half year follow-up. Based on multivariate analysis depression was an independent predictor of mortality. Only 25% of the patients with CHF and depression were on antidepressant medications. Gottlieb and colleagues reported a relatively small study of patients with congestive heart failure and depression comparing paroxetine (an SSRI) versus placebo during a 12-week randomized trial [56]. There was a reduction in the

BDI score below 10 in 69% of the patients on paroxetine and 25% of the patients on placebo. Patients with a response to paroxetine had higher general health scores and improvement in the Minnesota Living with Heart Failure questionnaire score. There were no adverse effects. This study would suggest that antidepressants from the SSRI drug group can work in patients with heart failure at least over relative short study periods. Jiang and co-workers have designed a larger randomized, double-blind controlled trial of sertraline versus placebo in patients with congestive heart failure in major depressive disorder [57]. This study will evaluate the effect of drug therapy on depression score and/or cardiovascular status. The results are not available yet.

Patients with ICDs frequently have an increase in psychiatric symptoms and diagnoses following implantation. Thomas, et al. monitored 57 patients who were participants in the SCD-HeFT study for depression, anxiety, and social support [58]. Thirty-five percent of these patients were depressed at the initial assessment. Patients receiving ICD shocks had an increased frequency of depression over time, and patients who did not receive ICD shocks had a decrease in depression. Forty-five percent of these patients had anxiety at initial evaluation. The shocks did not change the frequency of anxiety. Patients with New York Heart Association class III congestive heart failure tended to have decreased anxiety over time. Finally, these patients had poor social support. In younger patients this decreased over time, whereas in older patients it increased over time. Peterson, et al. have reviewed studies on psychological interventions following ICD implantation [59]. They concluded that cognitive behavioral therapy and structured exercise decreased anxiety in these patients. There was no major effect on depression, quality of life, and number of shocks.

There is little information on drug therapy in patients with anxiety and depression who have ICDs. SSRIs have a relatively benign cardiovascular adverse effect profile and do not significantly change heart rate, blood pressure, ejection fraction, or ectopy in these patients. Although these features are undoubtedly important in patients with ICDs and heart failure, these drugs have the potential to change the defibrillation threshold, the sensing of ventricular tachycardia, and the pacing threshold which makes antitachycardia pacing effective. Carnes, et al. reported a patient who was taking venlafaxine during the initial defibrillator testing [60]. This patient could not be internally defibrillated while on this medication but was internally defibrillated after the medication was discontinued. Venlafaxine has cardiac sodium channel blocker activity and potentially changed the defibrillation threshold. Other SSRIs may have similar activity, and it will be difficult to extrapolate from results from patients with congestive heart failure who are treated with drugs for depression to patients with congestive heart failure and ICDs. These patients should benefit from cognitive behavioral therapy which focuses on anxiety, apprehension, avoidance behavior, fear of shocks, and distorted cognition, and from stress management and structured exercise [61]. Patients with significant psychiatric disorders will need to be co-managed with psychiatrists with careful attention to the possibility of unexpected drug side effects if drugs are used.

Organized Protocol for Review of Patients Receiving ICD Shocks

Patients receiving one shock should call the cardiologist or electrophysio-logist and arrange follow-up [62]. Patients receiving more than one shock should go to an emergency department for an evaluation. The electrogram in the ICD memory should be reviewed to determine whether or not the patient had appropriate or inappropriate shocks. The clinician needs to determine the circumstances surrounding the shocks, in particular whether or not they occurred at rest or with physical activity. The physician needs to evaluate the patient for changes in clinical status, including myocardial ischemia, an increase in congestive heart failure, electrolyte abnormalities, or medication misadventures, including drug toxicity, drug interaction, and poor compliance. The electrophysiologist then needs to review device programming. Antitachycardia pacing is effective in as many as 90% of patients with ventricular tachycardia. This includes patients with both slow and fast tachycardia. If the patient has received inappropriate shocks then the discriminator algorithm should be reviewed to determine onset criteria, heart rate criteria, heart rhythm stability, and ventricular morphology. Changes in programming can potentially reduce inappropriate shocks. The electrophysiologist then needs to review the medication regimen. This patient should be on beta-blockers and ACE inhibitors, may require use of diuretics, and may benefit from aldosterone antagonists and statins. The addition of amiodarone represents a complex decision but has the potential to decrease the number of episodes of ventricular tachycardia, to reduce the rate of ventricular tachycardia, and to reduce the number of episodes of supraventricular tachycardia. However, amiodarone can increase defibrillation thresholds and slow the tachycardia rate below the device detection settings. This will require reprogramming by the electrophysiologist. These patients likely need additional education and/or counseling if they are having psychiatric symptoms such as anxiety, panic, and depression. They may benefit from referral to a psychiatrist or psychologist. Interventions could include cognitive behavioral therapy and/or anti-depressant medications. Serotonin re-uptake inhibitor medications likely have the safest side effect profile of antidepressant medicines, but the potential for toxicity and unexpected drug interactions should be considered. Patients with anxiety may benefit from benzodiazepines.

In summary, patients with heart failure and ICDs require a comprehensive management program with attention to LV function, arrthymias, and psychiatric syndromes. The use of ICDs actually increases the clinician's responsibility for comprehensive care.

CONCLUSION

ICD trials have provided important opportunities to improve the management and to prevent lethal ventricular arrhythmias. These trials have generated rich data bases which provide information about the natural history of advanced congestive heart failure and the benefit of organized chronic medical care with the use of beta-blockers and angiotensin converting inhibitors. These trials have also demonstrated that electric shocks have the potential to cause progression of congestive heart failure through myocardial dysfunction and possibly through complex interactions between the sympathetic nervous system and the central nervous system. These patients have a high incidence of psychiatric disorders and/or psychiatric symptoms which aggravate their underlying cardiac disease and reduce their quality of life. Psychiatric care has the potential to prolong life and to improve the quality of life in these patients.

REFERENCES

Moss, AJ; Hall, WJ; Cannom, DS; et al. Improved survival*N Engl J Med*, 1996, 335, 1933-40.

Moss, AJ; Zareba, W; Hall, WJ; et al. Prophylactic implantation of a defibrillator *N Engl J Med*, 2002, 346, 877-83.

Bardy, GH; Lee, KL; Mark, DB; et al. Amiodarone; Sudden Cardiac Death in Heart Failure Trial (SCD-HeFT) Investigators. In: N; Engl, J; Med.

2005, 352, 225-37. Erratum: *N Engl J Med*, 2005, 352, 2146.

ACC *Circulation*, 2006, 114, 385-484.

Tung, R; Zimetbaum, P; Josephson, ME. A critical appraisal of implantable cardioverter-defibrillator therapy for the prevention of sudden cardiac death. *J Am Coll Cardiol*, 2008, 52, 1111-1121.

Kadish, A; Dyer, A; Daubert, JP; et al. Defibrillators in Non-Ischemic Cardiomyopathy Treatment Evaluation (DEFINITE) Investigators Prophylactic defibrillator *N Engl J Med*, 2004, 350, 2151-8.

Daubert, JP; Zareba, W; Cannom, DS; *et al.* MADIT II Investigators. Inappropriate implantable cardioverter-defibrillator shocks in MADIT II: frequency, mechanisms, predictors, and survival impact. *J Am Coll Cardiol*, 2008, 51, 1357-65.

Poole, JE; Johnson, GW; Hellkamp, AS; et al. Prognostic importance of defibrillator shocks in patients with heart failure. *N Engl J Med*, 2008, 359, 1009-17.

Singer, I; Hutchins, GM; Mirowski, M; et al. Pathologic findings related to the lead system and repeated defibrillations in patients with the automatic implantable cardioverter-defibrillator. *J Am Coll Cardiol*, 1987, 10, 382-8.

Hasdemir, C; Shah, N; Rao, AP; et al. Analysis of troponin I levels after spontaneous implantable cardioverter defibrillator shocks. *J Cardiovasc Electrophysiol*, 2002, 13, 144-50.

Hurst, TM; Hinrichs, M; Breidenbach, C; et al. Detection of myocardial injury during transvenous implantation of automatic cardioverter-defibrillators. *J Am Coll Cardiol*, 1999, 34, 402-8.

Tokano, T; Bach, D; Chang, J; et al. Effect of ventricular shock strength on cardiac hemodynamics. *J Cardiovasc Electrophysiol*, 1998, 9, 791-7.

Bode, F; Wiegand, U; Raasch, W; et al. Differential effects of defibrillation, *Heart*, 1998, 79, 560-7.

Yu, JC; Lauer, MR; Young, C; et al. Ventricular pacing *Am Heart J*, 1996, 131, 1121-6.

Dougherty, CM. Psychological reactions and family adjustment in shock versus no shock groups after implantation of internal cardioverter defibrillator. *Heart Lung* 1995, 24, 281-291.

Ladwig, KH; Baumert, J; Marten-Mittag, B; et al. Posttraumatic stress symptoms and predicted mortality in patients with implantable cardioverter-defibrillators: results from the prospective living with an implanted cardioverter-defibrillator study. *Arch Gen Psychiatry*, 2008, 65, 1324-30.

Sears, SF; Jr; Conti, JB. Quality of life and psychological functioning of ICD patients. *Heart*, 2002, 87, 488-93.

Mark, DB; Anstrom, KJ; Sun; et al. *Sudden Cardiac Death in Heart*. Quality of life with defibrillator therapy or amiodarone in heart failure. *N Engl J Med*, 2008, 359, 999-1008.

Namerow, PB; Firth, BR; Heywood, GM; et al. Quality-of-life six months after CABG surgery in patients randomized to ICD versus no ICD therapy: findings from the CABG Patch Trial. *Pacing Clin Electrophysiol*, 1999, 22, 1305-13.

Huffman, JC; Smith, FA; Quinn, DK; et al. Post-MI psychiatric syndromes: six unanswered questions *Harv Rev Psychiatry*, 2006, 14, 305-18.

Kop, WJ; Gottdiener, JS; Tangen, CM; et al. Inflammation and coagulation factors in persons > 65 years of age with symptoms of depression but without evidence of myocardial ischemia. *Am J Cardiol.*, 2002, 89, 419-24.

Godemann, F; Butter, C; Lampe, F; et al. Panic disorders and agoraphobia *Clin Cardiol*, 2004, 27, 321-6.

Whang, W; Albert, CM; Sears, SF; Jr; et al. *TOVA Study Investigators*. Depression as a predictor for appropriate shocks among patients with implantable cardioverter-defibrillators: results from the Triggers of Ventricular Arrhythmias (TOVA) study. *J Am Coll Cardiol*, 2005, 45, 1090-5.

Wilkinson, DJ; Thompson, JM; Lambert, GW; et al. Sympathetic activity in patients with panic disorder at rest, under laboratory mental stress, and during panic attacks *Arch Gen Psychiatry*, 1998, 55, 511-20.

Alvarenga, ME; Richards, JC; Lambert, G; et al. Psychophysiological mechanisms in panic disorder: a correlative analysis of noradrenaline spillover, neuronal noradrenaline reuptake, power spectral analysis of heart rate variability, and psychological variables. *Psychosom Med*, 2006, 68, 8-16.

Fleet, R; Lespérance, F; Arsenault, A; et al. Myocardial perfusion study of panic attacks in patients with coronary artery disease. *Am J Cardiol*, 2005, 96, 1064-8.

Cevik, C; Perez-Verdia, A; Nugent, K. Implantable cardioverter defibrillators and their role in heart Europace 2009 Apr 8. [Epub ahead of print].

Bristow, MR; Saxon, LA; Boehmer, J; et al. Comparison of Medical Therapy, Pacing, and Defibrillation in Heart Failure (COMPANION) Investigators. Cardiac resynchronization therapy with or without an implantable defibrillator in advanced chronic heart failure. *N Engl J*

Med., 2004, 350, 2140-50.

Cevik, C; Perez-Verdia, A; Nugent, K. Prophylactic implantation of cardioverter-defibrillators in idiopathic nonischemic dilated cardiomyopathy for the primary prevention of death: A narrative review (unpublished data).

Desai, AS; Fang, JC; Maisel, WH; et al. Implantable defibrillators for the prevention of mortality in patients with nonischemic cardiomyopathy: a meta-analysis of randomized controlled trials. *JAMA*, 2004, 292, 2874-9.

Focused update incorporated into the ACC *J Am Coll Cardiol.*, 2009, 53, e1-e90.

Comparative effects of therapy with captopril and digoxin in patients with mild to moderate heart failure. *The Captopril-Digoxin Multicenter Research Group JAMA*, 1988, 259, 539-44.

Effect of enalapril on survival in patients with reduced left ventricular ejection fractions and congestive heart failure. The SOLVD Investigators. *N Engl J Med*, 1991, 325, 293-302.

Lubsen, J; Hoes, A; Grobbee, D. Implications of trial *Lancet*, 2000, 356, 1757-9.

Pfeffer, MA; Swedberg, K; Granger, CB; et al. Effects of candesartan on mortality *Lancet*, 2003, 362, 759-66.

Cohn, JN; Tognoni, G. A randomized trial of the angiotensin receptor blocker valsartan in chronic heart failure. *N Engl J Med*, 2001, 345, 1667-75.

Pitt, B; Zannad, F; Remme, WJ; et al. for the Randomized Aldactone Evaluation Study Investigators. The effect of spironolactone on morbidity and mortality in patients with severe heart failure. *N Engl J Med*, 1999, 341, 709-17.

Packer, M; Fowler, MB; Roecker, EB; et al. Effect of carvedilol on the morbidity of patients with severe chronic heart failure: results of the Carvedilol Prospective Randomized Cumulative Survival (COPERNICUS) study. *Circulation*, 2002, 106, 2194-2187.

Effect of metoprolol CR/XL in chronic heart failure: Metoprolol CR/XL Randomized Intervention Trial in Congestive Heart Failure (MERIT-HF). *Lancet.*, 1999, 353, 2001-7.

Wathen, MS; DeGroot, PJ; Sweeney, MO; et al. Prospective randomized multicenter trial of empirical antitachycardia pacing versus shocks for spontaneous rapid ventricular tachycardia in patients with implantable cardioverter-defibrillators: Pacing Fast Ventricular Tachycardia Reduces Shock Therapies (Pain FREE Rx II) trial results. *Circulation*, 2004, 110, 2591-6.

Schoels, W; Steinhaus, D; Johnson, WB; et al. Optimizing implantable cardioverter-defibrillator treatment of rapid ventricular tachycardia: antitachycardia pacing therapy during charging. *Heart Rhythm*, 2007, 4, 879-85.

Wilkoff, BL; Williamson, BD; Stern, RS; et al. PREPARE Study Investigators. Strategic programming of detection and therapy parameters in implantable cardioverter-defibrillators reduces shocks in primary prevention patients: results from the PREPARE (Primary Prevention Parameters Evaluation) study. *J Am Coll Cardiol*, 2008, 52, 541-50.

Schwab, JO; Gasparini, M; Lunati, M; et al. Avoid Delivering Therapies for Nonsustained Fast Ventricular Tachyarrhythmia in Patients with Implantable Cardioverter/Defibrillator: The ADVANCE III Trial. *J Cardiovasc Electrophysiol* 2009 Jan 9. [Epub ahead of print]

Reiter, MJ; Reiffel, JA. Importance of beta blockade in the therapy of serious ventricular arrhythmias *Am J Cardiol*, 1998, 82, 9I-19I.

Ellison, KE; Hafley, GE; Hickey, K; et al. Effect of beta-blocking therapy on outcome in the Multicenter UnSustained Tachycardia Trial (MUSTT) *Circulation*, 2002, 106, 2694-2699.

The Cardiac Arrhythmia Suppression Trial (CAST) Investigators. Preliminary report: effect of encainide and flecainide on mortality in a randomized trial of arrhythmia suppression after myocardial infarction. *N Engl J Med.*, 1989, 321, 406-12.

The Cardiac Arrhythmia Suppression Trial II Investigators. Effect of the antiarrhythmic agent moricizine on survival after myocardial infarction. *N Engl J Med.*, 1992, 327, 227-33.

Waldo, AL; Camm, AJ; deRuyter, H; et al. for the SWORD Investigators. Effect of d-sotalol on mortality in patients with left ventricular dysfunction after recent and remote myocardial infarction. Survival with Oral d-Sotalol. Lancet 1996, 348, 7-12. *Erratum in: Lancet*, 1996, 348, 416.

Pratt, CM; Camm, AJ; Cooper, W; et al. Mortality in the Survival with Oral D-sotalol (SWORD) trial: why did patients die? *Am J Cardiol*, 1998, 81, 869 -76.

Doval, HC; Nul, DR; Grancelli, HO; et al. for the Grupo de Estudiode la Sobrevida en la Insuficiencia Cardiaca en Argentina (GESICA). Randomised trial of low-dose amiodarone in severe congestive heart failure. *Lancet*, 1994, 344, 493-8.

Connolly, SJ. Meta-analysis of antiarrhythmic drug trials *Am J Cardiol*, 1999,

84, 90R-93R.

Farre, J; Romero, J; Rubio, JM; et al. Amiodarone and "primary" prevention of sudden death: critical review of a decade of clinical trials. *Am J Cardiol*, 1999, 83, 55D-63D.

Connolly, SJ; Dorian, P; Roberts, RS; et al. Comparison of B-Blockers, Amiodarone Plus B-Blockers, or Sotalol for Prevention of Shocks from Implantable Cardioverter Defibrillators. The OPTIC Study: A Randomized Trial. *JAMA*, 2006, 295, 165-171

Pacifico, A; Hohnloser, SH; Williams, JH; et al. Prevention of implantable-defibrillator shocks by treatment with sotalol. d, l-Sotalol Implantable Cardioverter-Defibrillator Study Group. *N Engl J Med*, 1999, 340, 1855-1862

O'Connor, CM; Jiang, W; Kuchibhatla, M; et al. Antidepressant use, depression *Arch Intern Med*, 2008, 168, 2232-7.

Gottlieb, S; Kop, W; Thomas, S; Katzen, S; et al. A double-blind placebo-controlled pilot study of controlled-release paroxetine on depression and quality of life in chronic heart failure. *Am Heart J*, 2007, 153, 868-873.

Jiang, W; O'Connor, C; Silva, SG; et al. SADHART-CHF. Safety and efficacy of sertraline for depression in patients with CHF (SADHART-CHF): a randomized, double-blind, placebo-controlled trial of sertraline for major depression with congestive heart failure. *Am Heart*, 2008, 156, 437-44.

Thomas, SA; Friedmann; Gottlieb, SS; et al. Sudden Cardiac Death in Heart. Changes in psychosocial distress in outpatients with heart failure with implantable cardioverter defibrillators. *Heart Lung.*, 2009, 38, 109-20.

Pedersen, SS; van den Broek, KC; Sears, SF; Jr. Psychological intervention *Pacing Clin Electrophysiol.*, 2007, 30, 1546-54.

Carnes, C; Pickworth, K; Votolato, N; et al. Elevated defibrillation threshold with venlafaxine therapy. *Pharmacotherapy*, 2004, 24, 1095-1098.

Kohn, CS; Petrucci, RJ; Baessler, C; et al. The effect of psychological intervention on patients' long-term adjustment to the ICD: a prospective study. *Pacing Clin Electrophysiol* 2000, 23, 450-6.

Gehi, AK; Mehta, D; Gomes, JA. Evaluation and management *JAMA*, 2006, 296, 2839-47.

In: Congestive Heart Failure...   ISBN: 978-1-60876-677-2
Editors: J. E. García et al. pp. 61-88   © 2010 Nova Science Publishers, Inc.

Chapter 3

REVERSIBLE LEFT VENTRICULAR DYSFUNCTION: THE TAKOTSUBO SYNDROME

Michael John Daly

Clinical Research Fellow
The Heart Centre, Royal Victoria Hospital,
Belfast, UK

ABSTRACT

Takotsubo cardiomyopathy, also called left ventricular apical ballooning syndrome or ampulla cardiomyopathy is a clinical entity first described by Dote *et al* in the Japanese population, particularly in post-menopausal women [1]. Since then, this unique type of reversible left ventricular dysfunction has been increasingly reported in the literature and has provoked intense debate regarding its aetiology, natural history, treatment and long-term outcome. Through improving our understanding of this modern cardiomyopathy, we hope to unlock the secrets of myocardial stunning and hibernation, in addition to how endogenous hormonal imbalances may affect and even "break" our hearts.

In this chapter, we aim to uncover the many hormonal influences on myocardial function and discuss possible aetiological mechanisms, diagnostic modalities and management strategies of the Takotsubo syndrome. Furthermore, we shall try to understand what this 'new' cardiomyopathy has to teach us in relation to the modern care and treatment of not only the cardiac patient, but all our patients.

INTRODUCTION

Takotsubo cardiomyopathy, otherwise known as transient left ventricular apical ballooning syndrome and ampulla or stress-induced cardiomyopathy is a modern phenomenon first described in the Japanese population by Dote *et al* [1]. This syndrome is characterized by a peculiar, yet distinctive regional systolic dysfunction of the left ventricular (LV) apex and mid-ventricle, with hyperkinesis of the basal LV segments. The shape of the LV at end-systole on ventriculography is reminiscent of a traditional ceramic octopus trap used in Japan, a so-called "tako-tsubo". Clinical presentation commonly resembles that of acute myocardial infarction with both chest pain and anterior ST-segment elevation being typical [2]. Pivotal to the diagnosis is an absence of obstructive coronary artery disease on angiography, and complete reversibility of left ventricular systolic impairment, with all other causes of reversible left ventricular dysfunction having been excluded (Table 1) [3].

Despite increasing reports, Takotsubo cardiomyopathy remains under-recognised and is often misdiagnosed. As an important differential diagnosis of acute myocardial infarction, distinguishing it from obstructive coronary artery disease by angiography is always indicated, since the differences in both long-term survival and overall cardiovascular morbidity are significant [4].

Epidemiology

The precise incidence of Takotsubo cardiomyopathy is unknown due to its novel nature, varied presentation and evolving diagnostic criteria [5]. However, several investigations in recent years have assessed the prevalence of Takotsubo cardiomyopathy in a variety of geographical populations [6 - 15]. Among patients presenting with symptoms and signs suggestive of acute coronary syndrome, the reported prevalence of Takotsubo cardiomyopathy ranges from 0.7 – 2.5% (Table 2) [2] with a gender-specific prevalence in women of 6 – 7.5% [12, 15]. All reports included in a recent meta-analysis describe a striking gender bias, with 90.7% (95% CI: 88.2 - 93.2%, range 69.2 - 100%) of all patients with the syndrome being female (mean age range 62 – 76 years) [2] and < 3% of all reported patients being < 50 years [16, 17]. The reason for the female predominance is currently unknown; however, consequently, speculation has arisen into endogenous estrogen depletion as an aetiological stimulus for the syndrome [18].

Table 1. Causes of reversible myocardial dysfunction encountered in clinical practice [3]

Afterload excess: aortic valve disease, severe hypertension
Electrolytes: hypocalcaemia, hypomagnesaemia, hypophosphataemia
Endocrine: phaeochromocytoma, thyrotoxicosis, hypothyroidism
Haemochromatosis
Inflammatory: acute myocarditis, cardiac transplant rejection
Nutritional deficiency: thiamine, selenium
Tachycardia-induced cardiomyopathy
Toxic exposure: alcohol, amphetamine, cocaine, interferon-α, scorpion venom

Table 2. Prevalence of Takotsubo Cardiomyopathy (TC) [2]

Reference	Country	Sample size	Prevalence of TC
Haghi et al. [6]	Germany	2031	2.5%
Bybee et al. [7]	USA	NR	2.2%
Ito et al. [8]	Japan	1023	1.5%
Akashi et al. [9]	Japan	637	1.9%
Matsuoka et al. [10]	Japan	450	2.2%
Schneider et al. [11]	Germany	1085	2.3%
Wedekind et al. [12]	Germany	215	2.3%
Parodi et al. [13]	Italy	1811	2.0%
Pillière et al. [14]	France	1613	0.7%
Elian et al. [15]	Israel	638	2.0%

Aetiology

The cause of Takotsubo cardiomyopathy remains unknown, however multiple aetiological theories exist. All available evidence is consistent with the concept that the syndrome results from extreme emotional (26-45%) and/or physiological stress (17-50%) [19]. A study of 107 North American patients suggests a preceding emotional/physical stressor in 72 (83%) patients with Takotsubo cardiomyopathy (Table 3) [20]. Additional physical causes such as renal colic, pulmonary embolism, pneumothorax, transient ischaemic attack and epilepsy have been noted in a small number of patients [4]. Recently, severe hyponatraemia in the absence of seizure activity has been postulated as a physiological precipitant of the syndrome [21]. Historically, hyponatraemia associated with complex endocrine disease or seizure activity has been associated with the development of Takotsubo cardiomyopathy [22], however intracellular calcium overload due to impaired function of the sodium-calcium pumps in the context of isolated hyponatraemia may have an aetiological role [23].

Table 3. Aetiological stimuli in Takotsubo Cardiomyopathy [20]

Emotional Stressors	**33%**
Worsening of psychiatric illness requiring hospitalization	8%
Prolonged argument	8%
Death of a close relative	6%
Recent diagnosis of cancer	4%
Panic attack	2%
Inability to meet office work deadlines	2%
Late for a meeting	1%
News of relative in road traffic accident	1%
Witnessing a road accident	1%
Physiological stressors	**50%**
Unaccustomed physical exertion	13%
Non-cardiac surgery or procedure	12%
COPD / Asthma exacerbation	7%
Recent hospitalization for a severe illness	3%
Recurrent severe epistaxis	3%
Uncomfortable exposure to high temperatures	3%
Angioedema /drug-induced hives	3%
Fractures	3%
Narcotic overdose	2%
Recurrent falls while at home	1%
No identifiable stressors	**17%**

One potential aetiological stimulus, occurring as a consequence of emotional and physical stress, is that of increased endogenous catecholamine production. Catecholamines are recognized as having a toxic effect on the myocardium, e.g. responsibility for the reversible ventricular dysfunction seen in phaeochromocytoma [24]. Increased catecholamine levels decrease the viability of myocytes through cyclic adenosine monophosphate (cAMP)-mediated calcium overload and are also a potential source of oxygen-derived free radicals that may cause myocyte injury. Free radicals can interfere with sodium and calcium transporters, resulting in myocyte dysfunction through increased trans-sarcolemmal calcium influx and cellular calcium overload [25].

Table 4. Clinical characteristics in 114 patients [20]

Female	106 (93%)
Body mass index (mean ± SD, kg/m^2)	26 ± 6
Diabetes mellitus	9 (8%)
Hypertension	75 (66%)
Hyperlipidaemia	38 (33%)
Smoker:	
Current	26 (23%)
Past	28 (24%)
Never	60 (53%)
Presenting sign or symptom:	
Chest pain	79 (69%)
Dyspnoea	20 (18%)
ECG abnormalities	7 (6%)
Syncope and other	8 (7%)

Depression is known to increase the incidence of coronary disease in patients with no apparent cardiac disease at the time of initial presentation [26]. Surveys indicate that 15.8% of postmenopausal women report depressed mood and 17.9% report either full-blown panic attacks or symptom-limited attacks [26, 27]. Epinephrine is released at rest and during spontaneous attacks in patients with panic disorder [28]. Radiotracer studies have shown reduced extraction of norepinephrine and epinephrine during cardiac transit in this group of patients [29]. This reduced reuptake has been attributed to impairment of the norepinephrine transporter, resulting in increased cardiac response to endogenous catecholamine surges [30]. Furthermore, studies in patients with panic attacks have demonstrated that induced panic attacks cause myocardial perfusion defects in patients with known coronary disease [31]. It has therefore been suggested that patients with Takotsubo cardiomyopathy have underlying psychiatric comorbidities, such as anxiety and/or panic attacks, and that these contribute to the pronounced cardiac syndrome during periods of acute stress [30].

Clinical Features

The clinical presentation of Takotsubo cardiomyopathy is indistinguishable from that of acute coronary syndrome in the majority of cases, with many patients having risk factors for atherosclerosis (Table 4) [20]. The most commonly reported presenting symptoms are chest pain (83.4%, 95% CI: 80.0 - 86.7%) and dyspnoea (20.4%, 95% CI: 16.3 - 24.5%) however, initial presentations with syncope and palpitations [9, 10, 14, 32 - 36], nausea and vomiting [9, 37], cardiogenic shock [38, 39], ventricular fibrillation [37] and cardiac arrest [36] have also been reported. In general, haemodynamic compromise is unusual, but mild to moderate congestive heart failure is frequent. Hypotension may occur due to either a reduction in stroke volume or dynamic left ventricular outflow tract obstruction [5].

Diagnosis

Laboratory Data

Cardiac Biomarkers

Mild elevation in cardiac enzymes have been reported in a number of cases [11, 12, 14, 35 - 43], with elevation in cardiac troponin T (cTnT) in 243 of 286 patients (85%, 95% CI: 80.8 - 89.1%) and elevation in creatinine kinase-MB (CK-MB) in 27 of 71 patients (38%, 95% CI: 26.7 - 49.3%) [2]. Patients with acute ST-elevation myocardial infarction (STEMI) have significantly higher levels of cTnT and CK-MB compared to those with Takotsubo cardiomyopathy (Table 5) [44]. In contrast, B-type natriuretic peptide (BNP) is significantly elevated in the acute phase ($\leq$ Day 2) of Takotsubo cardiomyopathy when compared to STEMI. Furthermore, the receiver-operator-characteristic (ROC) analyses suggest that both a BNP > 647 pg/ml (c-statistic = 0.84, sensitivity = 81%, specificity = 75%) and a ratio of BNP to peak (12-hour) cTnT > 502 (c-statistic = 0.95, sensitivity 94%, specificity 100%) reliably differentiate Takotsubo cardiomyopathy from STEMI [44].

Stress Hormones

Plasma catecholamines (epinephrine, norepinephrine and dopamine) are elevated in patients with Takotsubo cardiomyopathy at presentation ($\leq$ 2 days from symptom onset) and persist for 7 days after the initial event [39]. Plasma dihydroxyphenolglycol and dihydroxyphenylacetic acid, neuronal catecholamine metabolites, are significantly elevated on day three with plasma metanephrine, an extraneuronal catecholamine metabolite, becoming elevated on day seven. These elevations are significantly higher in those with Takotsubo cardiomyopathy when compared to a control population of patients with acute myocardial infarction and heart failure (Killip III myocardial infraction) [39]. Plasma levels of Neuropeptide-Y, which is stored with catecholamines in postganglionic sympathetic nerves and adrenal chromaffin cells and released during stress, is also significantly increased among patients with Takotsubo cardiomyopathy (186pg/ml (162 – 236 pg/ml) [normal range < 51pg/ml], $p < 0.01$) [39].

Electrocardiography

The most frequently encountered finding on admission electrocardiogram (ECG) is ST-segment elevation with subsequent development of T-wave inversion in the subacute phase [2]. ST-segment elevation occurs in 71.1% (95% CI: 67.2 - 75.1%) of patients and involves the praecordial leads (V_2-V_5) in 95.4% (95% CI: 92.6 - 98.2%) of cases. In 61.3% of patients, T-wave inversion is present on the initial ECG (95% CI: 56.7 - 65.9%). Patients with acute anterior STEMI however, exhibit a significantly greater extent of ST-segment elevation (STE) in all praecordial leads ($p < 0.05$) [45]. Regression portioning analysis by Bybee *et al* [45] indicates that the combination of STE < 1.75mm in lead V_2 in conjunction with STE < 2.5mm in lead V_3 is a reasonable simple predictor of Takotsubo cardiomyopathy (sensitivity 67%, specificity 94%). They suggest that the most discriminating combination of STE is identified by the formula:

$$STE\ [3V_2 + V_3 + 2V_5]$$

- using the optimal cut-off < 11.5mm, this formula discriminates between Takotsubo cardiomyopathy and acute anterior STEMI with a sensitivity of 94% and a specificity of 72% [45].

Transient prolongation of the QT_c interval is also consistently described in Takotsubo cardiomyopathy, with a median QT_c ranging from 445.8ms to

542ms [10, 37, 39, 46 - 49]. Mental stress and autonomic changes have been demonstrated to precipitate prolongation of ventricular repolarisation duration [50] and prolong the QT_c interval [51], respectively. During follow-up, complete normalization of repolarisation is observed at a mean time of 4 ± 2 months [52].

Table 5. Peak cardiac biomarker levels in Takotsubo cardiomyopathy (TC) and acute ST-elevation myocardial infarction (STEMI) [44]

	TC	STEMI	p-value
Troponin T (ng/ml) [§]	0.62 (0.18-0.84)	3.8 (2.04-6.57)	<0.0001
CK-MB (ng/ml) [¥]	10.1 (6.9-17.0)	96.7 (24.0-272.7)	0.0006
BNP (pg/ml) [Δ]	944 (650-2022)	206 (140-669)	0.009

§ - Normal range (NR) <0.01 ng/ml
¥ - NR ≤ 6.2 ng/ml
Δ - NR <350 pg/ml

In summary, electrocardiography does not allow reliable differentiation between Takotsubo cardiomyopathy and acute anterior STEMI with enough certainty to preclude the need for angiography, despite the above-mentioned subtle ECG differences.

Echocardiography

During the acute phase, all patients show a typical apical ballooning pattern with akinesia involving the apex, mid-distal septum and mid-distal anterolateral walls as well as hypercontractile basal segments (Figure 1) [19]. Mean left ventricular ejection fraction (LVEF) at presentation has been reported as $47 \pm 7\%$, with mean left ventricular end-diastolic volume (LVEDV) and left ventricular end-systolic volume (LVESV) being 107 ± 36ml and 58 ± 22ml respectively [52]. Both LVEDV and LVESV reduce significantly at hospital discharge and two-month follow-up (p<0.05) [52] with an increase in left ventricular systolic function at short-term follow-up (median: 20days), i.e. LVEF $58.8 \pm 9.5\%$ [53]. Left ventricular posterior wall thickness reduces significantly from 12.4 ± 1.8mm at baseline to 10.9 ± 0.9mm at long-term (≥ 62 days) follow-up (p = 0.003), with a reduction in end-diastolic interventricular septum diameter from 13.0 ± 2.1mm to $11.5 \pm$

2.2mm over the same time period (p = 0.026) [53]. The cause of this acute left ventricular hypertrophy remains unknown. Initial dynamic left ventricular outflow tract obstruction has been related to a moderate ventricular hypertrophy, hypercontractility of the basal segments and systolic anterior motion (SAM) of the mitral valve. Furthermore, SAM-phenomenon has been implicated as an important factor in the development of apical ballooning [54]. The presence of mild/moderate mitral and tricuspid regurgitation at baseline, without left ventricular or mitral annular dilatation, which has regressed at long-term follow-up, has recently been described [54]. In addition, transient pulmonary hypertension develops in some patients in response to an elevation in left atrial pressure with or without significant mitral regurgitation. Right ventricular involvement is rarely described in the literature [20, 55, 56].

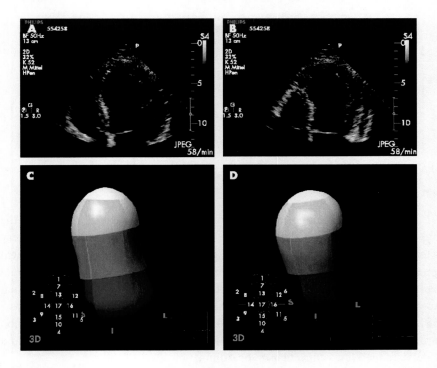

Figure 1. Transthoracic echocardiogram showing four-chamber views during diastole (A) and systole (B) in a patient presenting with Takotsubo cardiomyopathy. Real time three-dimensional echocardiography shows the typical contractile pattern of Takotsubo cardiomyopathy with akinesia of apical segments and hypercontractility of the basal segments (diastole C; systole D). Reproduced with permission from Nef *et al.* [19]

Coronary Angiography and Ventriculography

Most patients with Takotsubo cardiomyopathy have angiographically normal coronary arteries or mild atherosclerosis. Normal coronary arteries are reported in 88% patients (95% CI: 83.8 - 92.0%) with Takotsubo cardiomyopathy, with the remainder (12%) having non-critical luminal stenoses [2]. Obstructive coronary disease may rarely coexist by virtue of its prevalence in the population at risk. Recent reports suggest evidence of microvascular dysfunction in patients with Takotsubo syndrome. Two studies [7, 57] have demonstrated abnormal thrombolysis in myocardial infarction (TIMI) frame counts in all coronary arteries reflecting reduced coronary blood flow (Table 6) [52]. Ventriculography usually displays typical apical ballooning and a hypercontraction of the basal segments.

Table 6. TIMI flow grade and corrected TIMI frame count in the three coronary arteries [52]

	RCA	LCX	LAD
TIMI flow grade 2 (% pts)	33	33	72
Abnormal (>27frames) CTFC (% pts)	41	71	55
Mean CTFC (frames)	29 ± 16	33 ± 13	29 ± 13

Abbreviations: CTFC = corrected TIMI frame count; RCA = right coronary artery; LCX = left circumflex artery; LAD = left anterior descending artery.

It as also been suggested that a disrupted atherosclerotic plaque in the mid-portion of a long left anterior descending (LAD) coronary artery extending along the diaphragmatic LV aspect could account for the typical appearance on ventriculography (Figure 2). The disruption of a plaque could lead to an acute coronary syndrome with early reperfusion, and thus minimal enzymatic release, resulting in left ventricular stunning rather than necrosis [58]. It has therefore been hypothesized that in some patients with Takotsubo cardiomyopathy, the underlying cause is an ACS with early reperfusion and widely stunned left ventricular myocardium.

However, the majority of patients presenting with transient left ventricular apical ballooning syndrome do not have a long recurrent distal LAD on angiography [59]. More recently, atypical forms of Takotsubo cardiomyopathy with variant distributions of wall motion abnormalities and several unusual features have increasingly been reported, including transient mid-ventricular ballooning with apical and basal hyperkinesis, patients presenting with features of left ventricular non-compaction or patients with small areas of necrosis [60 - 63]. In patients with this atypical apical ballooning a different distribution of the adrenergic receptors might be hypothesized, as it seems difficult to relate the transient mid-ventricular dysfunction to an ischaemic event [61, 64].

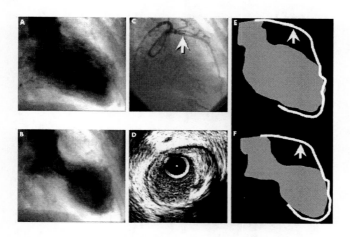

Figure 2. (A) End-diastolic frame of the left ventriculogram. (B) End-systolic frame of the left ventriculogram. (C) RAO 30° projection of the left coronary artery; the arrow shows the IVUS transducer placement. (D) Cross-sectional IVUS view of the LAD, showing a disrupted eccentric plaque with positive remodeling from 12 to 5 o'clock. At 4 o'clock there is an image of ulceration, with a cavity inside the plaque. The cavity is located just beside a calcification zone (acoustic shadow from 4 to 6 o'clock). Panels E (diastole) and F (systole) are a schematic representation of the LAD and LV; the arrow shows the ruptured plaque location. Note that the akinetic area corresponds to the LV area between the plaque and the end of the LAD. Reproduced with permission from Ibanez *et al* [62].

Cardiovascular magnetic resonance imaging

Cardiovascular magnetic resonance (CMR) imaging provides precise morphologic and functional information on the left ventricle (Figure 3) [19]. CMR has been performed prospectively in three studies on Takotsubo cardiomyopathy [35, 65, 66]. In contrast to the typical features of acute myocardial infarction or myocarditis, almost all patients show no delayed gadolinium hyperenhancement, consistent with viable myocardium [2]. To date, only three cases of delayed hyperenhancement have been reported [19].

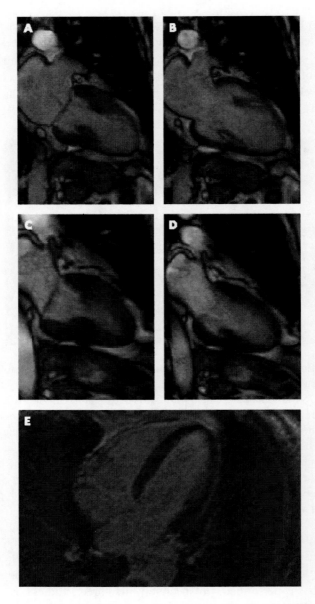

Figure 3. Cine sequences of cardiac magnetic resonance imaging during systole (A) and diastole (B) in the acute phase. Normal function could be documented after 3 weeks (systole, C; diastole, D). Late enhancement does not show any increased signal intensity (E). Reproduced with permission from Nef *et al* [19].

In all cases, the observed endocardial delayed hyperenhancement is small in comparison to the extent of wall motion abnormality. Since areas of hyperenhancement originate from the epicardium in myocarditis, late enhancement sequences can assist in the differential diagnosis of Takotsubo cardiomyopathy. In addition, regional wall motion abnormalities of the right ventricle in the acute phase of the Takotsubo syndrome have recently been described [6].

Myocardial Single Photon Emission Computed Tomography

Several reports advocate myocardial single photon emission computed tomography (SPECT) to assess myocardial perfusion, fatty acid metabolism and sympathetic function in patients with Takotsubo cardiomyopathy (Figure 4) [38]. Reduced Technetium-99m tetrofosmin uptake indicating decreased myocardial perfusion is observed during the acute phase [8, 38, 45], which recovers after 3 - 5days. Abnormal fatty acid metabolism reflecting myocardial ischaemia using iodine-123-beta-methyl-p-iodophenyl pentadecanoic acid (^{123}I-BMIPP) is also demonstrated during the acute phase [8, 38, 67]. In addition, decreased myocardial ^{123} I-MIBG uptake indicating sympathetic nerve dysfunction has also been reported [8, 38, 68]. These findings support the hypothesis of myocardial stunning as a pathophysiological mechanism.

Endomyocardial Biopsies

Endomyocardial biopsies have been performed in a subset of patients with Takotsubo cardiomyopathy [39, 41, 45, 58, 69]. Interstitial fibrosis, mild cell vacuolation, intracytoplasmic glycogen deposition [70] as well as focal myocardial depletion and contraction-band necrosis have been described [2]. No evidence of myocarditis has been found on biopsy and viral antibody titres have been negative throughout.

Typically, myocytes are hypertrophied (> 20μm) and of varied size. PAS staining of acute biopsies reveals large areas of intracytoplasmic glycogen, with a significant reduction in 'recovered' biopsies [70]. In electron microscopy, the main alteration observed in the acute phase includes numerous vacuoles of differing size and content leading to an enlarged myocyte diameter. The specific arrangement of cytoskeletal and contractile proteins is dissolved, with sporadic contraction bands. In addition, the interstitial space is widened and contains fibrotic material including collagen fibrils, formations of cell debris, macrophages and an increased number of

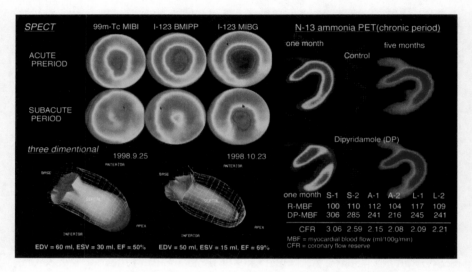

Figure 4. Nuclear cardiographic evaluations showing marked perfusion (^{99m}Tc-sestamibi [MIBI]) metabolic (^{123}I-BMIPP or ^{123}I-MIBG) mismatches mainly at the left ventricular apex. However, in the subacute period, this perfusion metabolic mismatch decreased after the functional recovery (three-dimensional left ventriculography by ^{99m}Tc-MIBI). After 5-months, PET by ^{13}N-ammonia showed improvement in the coronary flow reserve assessed by dipyridamole administration. EDV = end-diastolic volume; EF = ejection fraction; ESV = end-systolic volume; MBF = myocardial blood flow. Reproduced with permission from Tsuchihashi et al [38].

fibroblasts. The myocytes in the 'recovered' biopsies show a normal size, only a few small vacuoles, a normal rearrangement of the intracellular structures and a regular composition of the myocardium (Figure 5) [70]. Immunohistochemistry of intracellular proteins actin, dystrophin and connexin-43 reveals significant differences between 'acute' and 'recovered' biopsies (Figure 6). These findings correspond with the typical histological signs of catecholamine toxicity, which are described as focal mononuclear inflammation, areas of fibrotic response and characteristic contraction bands [71]. Contraction bands have been reported in several clinical settings of extensive catecholamine production, such as phaeochromocytoma [72] and subarachnoid haemorrhage [73], showing that catecholamines may be an important link between emotional stress and cardiac injury [39].

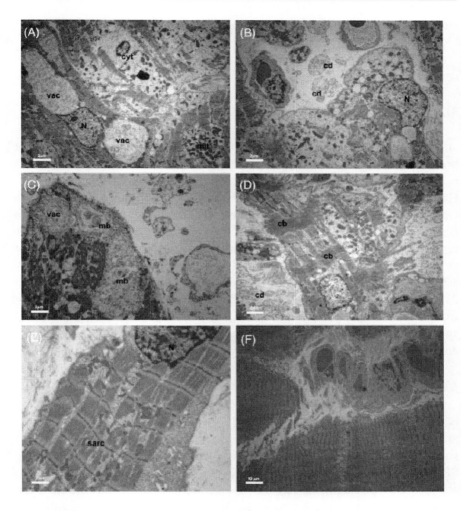

Figure 5. Electron microscopy of 'acute' biopsies showing numerous vacuoles of different sizes and contents (myelin bodies, residual cellular products), loss of contractile material, and areas of non-specified cytoplasm (A). The interstitial space is widened containing formation of cellular debris (B). In the 'acute' phase, formation of myelin bodies could be documented (C). In Takotsubo cardiomyopathy contraction bands of sarcomeres were found (D). 'Recovered' biopsies show a nearly complete rearrangement of contractile material with regularly distributed sarcomeres, normal nuclei and mitochondria (E, F). vac, vacuole; svac, small vacuole; N, nucleus; cyt, cytoplasm; mit, mitochondria; cd, cellular debris; mb, myelin bodies; sarc, sarcomeres; cb, contraction band. Reproduced with permission from Nef *et al* [70].

Pathophysiological Mechanisms

Several pathophysiological concepts have been proposed for Takotsubo cardiomyopathy, however the precise underlying mechanism remains unclear.

Multivessel Epicardial Coronary Artery Spasm

As previously discussed, invariably all patients have either angiographically normal coronary arteries or non-obstructive disease at presentation. It is therefore not surprising that epimyocardial vasospasm has been proposed as responsible for inducing ischaemia in these patients. However, in argument with this hypothesis is the reality that, except in rare cases [62], the region of wall motion abnormality (LV apex) does not correspond to the perfusion territory of a single coronary artery, rather represents a confluence of coronary arterial perfusion [19]. Provocation of coronary artery vasospasms by either acetylcholine or ergovine has been assessed [9, 32, 33 38, 40 - 1, 45, 48, 69] and been shown to collectively affect 27.6% of patients (95% CI: 19.7 - 35.5%) with variable frequency ranging from 0 to 71.4% [2]. Gianni *et al* found that only 1.4% of patients experienced spontaneous multivessel epicardial spasm [17]. Taken together, multivessel epicardial spasm seems to be an unlikely mechanism.

Coronary Microvascular Impairment

Microvascular dysfunction in the absence of obstructive coronary disease is demonstrated by TIMI frame counts [7, 57] and TIMI myocardial perfusion grades [36]. Decreased coronary flow velocity reserve by Doppler guidewire [74] and decreased myocardial perfusion by ^{99m}Tc-tetrofosmin myocardial SPECT [8, 38, 45] are also in favor of this hypothesis. In addition, myocardial contrast echocardiographic studies reveal perfusion defects in the apex returning to a homogeneous signal after one-month follow-up, suggesting that microvascular dysfunction might be responsible for the reversible contractile impairment [75]. It remains unclear, however, whether coronary microvascular dysfunction is the primary mechanism involved in the pathogenesis of the syndrome or whether it is simply an associated secondary phenomenon, i.e. that myocardial stunning secondary to catecholamine-mediated microvascular dysfunction be a likely explanation for Takotsubo cardiomyopathy.

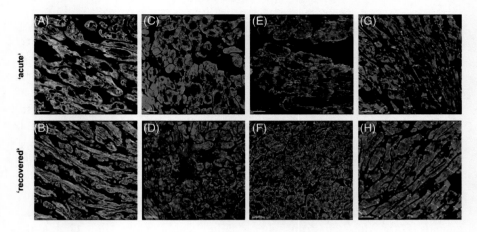

Figure 6.Immunohistochemistry of intracellular proteins (specific labeling green, phalloidin red, nuclei blue). α-actinin was detected only in the border zone during Takotsubo cardiomyopathy (TC) (A). After functional recovery a regular distribution was found (B). N-terminal dystrophin showed a decrease in TC verifying a loss of protein-to-protein interaction (C) in comparison with biopsies after functional recovery (D). C-terminal dystropin was unaltered in TC suggesting that integrity of the sarcolemma is maintained (E, F). Connexin-43 showed a reduced cell-cell connection in TC (G), whereas a myocardial integrity was documented after functional recovery (H). Reproduced with permission from Nef *et al* [70].

Catecholamine Cardiotoxicity

In addition to the putative role of catecholamines in triggering the inflammatory response, a direct myocardial or vascular toxic effect of catecholamines has been proposed to account for the pathophysiology of Takotsubo cardiomyopathy [70]. Catecholamine-mediated neurogenic myocardial stunning provoked by emotional or physiological stress is supported by both elevated plasma catecholamine measurements during the acute phase in more than 70% of patients [2] and evidence of sympathetic nerve hyperactivity demonstrated by SPECT using [123]I – MIBG, the radioiodinated analog for norepinephrine [8, 38, 68]. A recent study investigating direct catecholamine-induced myocyte injury found that acute β-adrenergic overload produces myocyte damage through calcium leakage while cardiac stem cells are spared, raising the question whether cardiac stem cell activation contributes to the rapid clinical recovery [76]. In addition, it has been suggested that the ensuing elevation in intracellular calcium concentration produces the ventricular dysfunction seen in catecholamine cardiotoxicity [78].

Circulating epinephrine exerts a much more potent hormonal effect on the heart than norepinephrine [79]. Takotsubo cardiomyopathy could therefore represent epinephrine-induced toxicity. Concurrent cardiac neuronal and adreno-medullary hormonal stimulation may occur, and this combination is well known to accompany emotional distress. It has been hypothesized that high plasma epinephrine levels trigger a switch in the cardiomyocyte intracellular signaling, after occupation of β_2-adrenoreceptors, from G_s protein to G_i protein coupling [80]. Furthermore, apical ballooning can be induced in a rat model of emotional stress and is prevented with combined α-adrenoreceptor and β-adrenoreceptor blockade [81].

The myocardial histological changes in Takotsubo cardiomyopathy resemble those seen in catecholamine cardiotoxicity in both animals [77] and humans [78]. Although diffuse heart failure can produce high circulating catecholamine concentrations, the attained levels are not as high as in Takotsubo cardiomyopathy and by definition would not explain the apical ballooning pattern.

Left ventricular outflow tract obstruction has been observed in patients with Takotsubo cardiomyopathy [82]. It has been hypothesized that, in the presence of elevated plasma catecholamines caused by emotional stress, mid-ventricular septal thickening leads to the transient severe mid-cavity obstruction, resulting in subendocardial ischaemia unrelated to a specific coronary artery territory [19]. However, it remains unclear whether the observed intraventricular gradient is a consequence rather than a cause of Takotsubo cardiomyopathy.

Therepeutic Options

Patients with Takotsubo cardiomyopathy generally recover spontaneously, however approximately 40% of patients develop congestive heart failure and a minority (~10%) develop acute cardiogenic shock or major haemodynamic compromise [4]. Other complications include life-threatening arrhythmias: third-degree atrioventricular block, ventricular tachycardia, ventricular fibrillation and cardiac arrest. Isolated cases of intramural thrombus with systemic emboli and left ventricular free-wall rupture have been reported [2].

There are no specific treatments for Takotsubo cardiomyopathy since the left ventricular function resolves spontaneously within weeks, however patients should be evaluated and initially treated in a manner similar to patients with acute myocardial infarction. When cardiogenic shock occurs, intra-aortic balloon pumping is well established in providing additional haemodynamic support [9]. As catecholamines could have a causative role in Takotsubo cardiomyopathy, therapy with epinephrine, ionotropic agents such as dobutamine, or both might lead to worsening of the condition, although in the absence of clinical studies this is a theoretical concern [84]. Data from an animal-model of Takotsubo cardiomyopathy suggest that its development seems to be diminished after α- and β-blockade [83]. However, it should be remembered that β-blockade may prolong an already prolonged QT_c interval and leave unopposed the potentially adverse effects of high concentrations of catecholamines at α-adrenoceptors [79]. Thus combined α- and β-blockade, such as labetalol, should be given in the acute phase and may prevent syndrome recurrence [19]. In general, given the possible pathophysiological mechanism of catecholamine-mediated myocardial stunning, long-term treatment with β-blockade may be an appropriate approach [2].

Thrombosis is often encountered in Takotsubo cardiomyopathy [85], which might reflect the vasoconstrictor, platelet activation, or prothombotic effects of extremely high circulating epinephrine levels [79]. Anticoagulation remains controversial, given the small risk of left ventricular free-wall rupture in these patients, however in order to prevent left ventricular thrombus formation administration of low molecular weight heparin is warranted [19]. After recovery of systolic contractile function, further anticoagulation with warfarin is not required. It should be remembered that epinephrine promotes platelet activation by stimulating platelet $α_2$ adrenoceptors, providing additional rationale for treatment with a combined α- and β-antagonist [79].

In the setting of life-threatening arrhythmias (torsades de pointes, ventricular fibrillation) the implantation of a cardioverter-defibrillator has to be considered [79].

Interest has emerged into estrogen supplementation as a potential therapy, given its prevention of Takotsubo cardiomyopathy in rats, however clinical trials have yet to be performed [79].

Prognosis

Takotsubo cardiomyopathy has an in-hospital mortality of 1.7% (95% CI: 0.5 - 2.8%) generally due to cardiac arrhythmia [4], with a more favorable outcome once recovered from the acute phase of the syndrome. It has been suggested that contrast-enhanced CMR be carried out after the acute-phase, since the presence of minor necrotic changes may imply an increased risk of cardiac arrhythmia in these patients, however it does not confer additional prognostic information [86]. Complete recovery is experienced by 96% of patients (95% CI: 93.8 - 98.1%) with recurrence being rarely reported (3.1%, 95% CI: 0.4 - 5.7%) [2]. Recurrence rate is highest within the first 4 years (2.9% per year), subsequently decreasing to 1.3% per year thereafter [4]. Importantly, the overall four-year survival and cardiovascular survival of patients with Takotsubo cardiomyopathy is similar to the expected survival for an age-, gender- and race-matched population [4]. However, morbidity within this time-period is significant, with almost one-third of patients continuing to have episodes of chest pain and one-third of these patients requiring hospital admission where coronary angiography is invariably normal. In summary, the four-year prognosis for patients with Takotsubo cardiomyopathy remains excellent.

CONCLUSION

Takotsubo cardiomyopathy represents a novel form of reversible left ventricular systolic dysfunction that is precipitated by sudden emotional or physiological stress. Aetiological mechanisms are probably complex and the brief summary outlined in this chapter represents only the beginning of our understanding of this neurocardiological condition. Given that abnormal catecholamine dynamics may cause Takotsubo cardiomyopathy, combined α- and β-blockade may mitigate the syndrome and estrogen supplementation may prevent it in the most at-risk population, post-menopausal women. It should however be considered in any patient presenting with symptoms and signs of an acute coronary syndrome, and as a cause of sudden cardiac death in those with no known history of heart disease. Overall, the prognosis is excellent in those who survive beyond the acute period without complication.

REFERENCES

[1]   Dote, K; Sato, H; Tateishi, H; Uchida, T; Ishihara, M. Myocardial stunning due to simultaneous multivessel coronary spasm: a review of 5 cases. *J Cardiol,* 1991, 21, 203-14.

[2]   Pilgrim, TM; Wyss, TR. Takotsubo cardiomyopathy or transient left ventricular apical ballooning syndrome: a systematic review. *Int J Cardiol,* 2008, 124, 283-92.

[3]   Daly, MJ; Dixon, LJ. Takotsubo cardiomyopathy presenting with acute pulmonary oedema. *Congest Heart Fail,* 2009, 15(1), 46-8.

[4]   Elesber, AA; Prasad, A; Lennon, RJ; Wright, RS; Lerman, A; Rihal, CS. Four-year recurrence rate and prognosis of the apical ballooning syndrome. *J Am Coll Cardiol,* 2007, 50(5), 448-52.

[5]   Prasad, A; Lerman, A; Rihal, CS. Apical ballooning syndrome (Tako-Tsubo or stress cardiomyopathy): a mimic of acute myocardial infarction. *Circulation,* 2008, 155(3), 408-17.

[6]   Haghi, D; Athanasiadis, A; Papavassiliu, T; et al. Right ventricular involvement in takotsubo cardiomyopathy. *Eur Heart J,* 2006, 27, 2433-9.

[7]   Bybee, KA; Prasad, A; Barsness, GW, et al. Clinical characteristics and thrombolysis in myocardial frame counts in women with transient left ventricular apical ballooning syndrome. *Am J Cardiol,* 2004, 94, 343-6

[8]   Ito, K; Sugihara, H; Kinoshita, N; Azuma, A; Matsubara, H. Assessment of takotsubo cardiomyopathy (transient left ventricular apical ballooning) using ^{99m}Tc-tetrofosmin, ^{123}I-BMIPP, ^{123}I-MIBG and ^{99m}Tc-PYP myocardial SPECT *Ann Nucl Med,* 2005, 19, 435-45.

[9]   Akashi, YJ; Musha, H; Kida, K, et al. Reversible ventricular dysfunction takotsubo cardiomyopathy. *Eur J Heart Fail,* 2005, 7, 1171-6.

[10]   Matsuoka, K; Okubo, S; Fujii, E, et al. Evaluation of the arrhythmogenicity of stress-induced "takotsubo cardiomyopathy" from the time course of the 12-lead surface electrocardiogram. *Am J Cardiol,* 2003, 92, 230-3.

[11]   Schneider, B; Stein, J. Tako-tsubo-like transient left ventricular dysfunction: prevalence and clinical findings in a western population. *Circulation,* 2004, 110, Suppl III, III-697.

[12]   Wedekind, H; Möller, K; Scholz, KH. Tako-Tsubo-Kardiomyopathie. *Herz,* 2006, 31(4), 339-46 [German].

[13]   Parodi, G; Del Pace, S; Carrabba, N. et al Incidence, clinical findings and outcome of women with left ventricular apical ballooning syndrome. *Am J Cardiol,* 2007, 99, 182-5.

[14]   Pillière, R, Mansencal, N; Digne, F; Lacombe, P; Joseph, T; Dubourg, O. Prevalence of tako-tsubo syndrome in a large urban agglomeration. *Am J Cardiol,* 2006, 98(5), 662-5.

[15] Elian, D; Osherov, A; Matetyky, S. et al. Left ventricular apical ballooning: not an uncommon variant of acute myocardial infarction in women. *Clin Cardiol,* 2006, 29, 9-12.

[16] Bybee, KA; Kara, T; Prasad, A; et al. Transient left ventricular apical ballooning syndrome; a mimic of ST-segment elevation myocardial infarction. *Ann Intern Med,* 2004, 141, 858-65.

[17] Gianni, M; Dentali, F; Grandi, AM. et al. Apical ballooning syndrome or Takotsubo cardiomyopathy: a systematic review. *Eur Heart J,* 2006, 27, 1523-9.

[18] Komesaroff, PA; Esler, MD; Sudhir, K. Estrogen supplementation attenuates glucocorticoid and catecholamine responses to mental stress in perimenopausal women. *J Clin Endocrinol Metab,* 1999, 84(2), 606-10.

[19] Nef, HM; Möllmann, H; Elsässer A. Tako-Tsubo cardiomyopathy (apical ballooning). *Heart* 2007, 93, 1309-15.

[20] Singh, NK; Rumman, S; Mikell, FL; Nallamothu, N; Rangaswamy, C. Stress cardiomyopathy: clinical and ventriculographic characteristics in 107 North American subjects. *Int J Cardiol,* 2009, In Press.

[21] AbouEzzeddine, O; Prasad, A. Apical ballooning syndrome precipitated by hyponatraemia. *Int J Cardiol,* 2009, In Press.

[22] Oki, K; Matsuura, W; Koide, J; Saito, Y; Ono, Y; Yanagihara, K. Ampulla cardiomyopathy associated with adrenal insufficiency and hypothyroidism. *Int J Cardiol,* 2006, 108(3), 391-2.

[23] Kolar, F; Cole, WC; Ostadal, B; Dhalla, NS. Transient ionotropic effects of low extracellular sodium in perfused rat heart. *Am J Physiol Sep* 1990, 259(3pt2), H712-9.

[24] Yamanaka, O; Yasumasa, F; Nakamura, T; Ohno, A; Endo, Y; Yoshimi, K; Miura, K; Yamaguchi, H. "Myocardial stunning"-like phenomenon during a crisis of phaeochromocytomas. *Jpn Circ J,* 1994, 58, 737-42.

[25] Daly, MJ; Dixon, LJ. Takotsubo cardiomyopathy in two preoperative patients with pain. *Anesth Analg,* 2009, In Press.

[26] Wassertheil-Smoller, S; Shumaker, S; Ockene, J. et al. Depression and cardiovascular sequelae in postmenopausal women. *Arch Intern Med,* 2004, 164, 289-98.

[27] Smoller, JW; Pollack, MH; Wassertheil-Smoller, S. et al. Prevalence and correlated of panic attacks in postmenopausal women. *Arch Intern Med,* 2003, 163, 2041-50.

[28] Wilkinson, DJ; Thompson, MJ; Lambert, GW. et al. Sympathetic activity in patients with panic disorder at rest, under laboratory mental stress, and during panic attacks. *Arch Gen Psychiatry,* 1998, 55, 511-20.

[29] Alvarenga, ME; Richards, JC; Lambert, G. et al. Psychophysiological mechanisms in panic disorder: a correlative analysis of noradrenaline spillover, neuronal noradrenaline reuptake, power spectral analysis of heart rate variability, and psychological variables. *Psychosom Med,* 2006, 68, 8-16.

[30] Nguyen, SB; Cevik, C; Otahbachi, M; Kumar, A; Jenkins, LA; Nugent, K. Do comorbid psychiatric disorders contribute to the pathogenesis of Tako-tsubo syndrome? A review of pathogenesis. *Congest Heart Fail,* 2009, 15(1), 31-4.

[31] Fleet, R; Lesperance, F; Arsenault, A, et al. Myocardial perfusion study of panic attacks in patients with coronary artery disease. *Am J Cardiol,* 2005, 96, 1064-8.

[32] Kawai, S; Suzuki, H; Yamaguchi, H; Tanaka, K; Sawada, H; Aizawa, T. et al. Ampulla cardiomyopathy ("takotsubo" cardiomyopathy)-reversible left ventricular dysfunction with ST segment elevation. *Jpn Circ J,* 2000, 64, 156-9.

[33] Ito, K; Sugihara, H; Azuma, A; Nakagawa, M. Assessment of takotsubo (ampulla) cardiomyopathy using [99m] Tc-tetrofosmin myocardial SPECT – comparison with acute cardiac syndrome. *Ann Nucl Med,* 2003, 17, 115-22.

[34] Lipiecki, J; Durel, N; Decalf, V. et al. Transient ballooning of the left ventricular apex, 10 new cases of tako-tsubo syndrome. *Arch Mal Coeur Vaiss,* 2005, 98(4), 275-80.

[35] Ibanez, B; Navarro, F; Farré, J. et al. Tako-tsubo transient left ventricular apical ballooning is associated with left anterior descending coronary artery with a long course along the apical diaphragmatic surface of the left ventricle. *Rev Esp Cardiol,* 2004, 57, 209-16.

[36] Elsber, A; Lerman, A; Bybee, KA. et al. Myocardial perfusion in apical ballooning syndrome correlates of myocardial injury. *Am Heart J* 2006, 152(3), 469.e9-13.

[37] Desmet, WJ; Adriaenssen, BF; Dens JA. Apical ballooning of the left ventricle: first series in white patients. *Heart,* 2003, 89, 1027-31.

[38] Tsuchuhashi, K; Ueshima, K; Uchida, T; Oh-mura, N; Kimura, K; Owa, M. et al. Transient left ventricular apical ballooning without coronary artery stenoses: a novel heart syndrome mimicking acute myocardial

infraction. Angina pectoris–myocardial infarction investigations in Japan. *J Am Coll Cardiol,* 2001, 38, 11-8.

[39] Wittstein, IS; Thiemann, DR; Lima, JA; Baughman, KL; Schulman, SP; Gerstenblith, G; Wu, KC; Rade, JJ; Bivalacqua, TJ; Champion, HC. Neurohumeral features of myocardial stunning due to sudden emotional stress. *N Engl J Med,* 2005, 352, 539-48.

[40] Sato, M; Fujita, S; Saito, A. et al. Increased incidence of transient left ventricular apical ballooning (so-called "takotsubo" cardiomyopathy) after the mid-Niigata prefecture earthquake. *Circ J,* 2006, 70, 947-53.

[41] Athanasiadis, A; Vogelsberg, H; Hauer, B; Meinhardt, G; Hill, S; Sechtem, U. Transient left ventricular dysfunction with apical ballooning (takotsubo cardiomyopathy) in Germany. *Clin Res Cardiol,* 2006, 95, 321-8.

[42] Hertting, K; Krause, K; Härle, T; Boczor, S; Reimers, J; Kuck, KH. Transient left ventricular apical ballooning in a community hospital in Germany. *Int J Cardiol,* 2006, 112(3), 282-8.

[43] El Mahmoud, R; Leyer, F; Michaud, O; Nallet, S; Cattan, S. Transient left ventricular apical ballooning syndrome or takotsubo cardiomyopathy. About 11 cases. *Ann Cardiol Angeiol,* 2006, 55(4), 210-5.

[44] Madhavan, M; Borlaug, BA; Lerman, A; Rihal, CS; Prasad, A. Stress hormone and circulating biomarker profile of apical ballooning syndrome (takotsubo cardiomyopathy): Insights into the clinical significance of BNP and Troponin levels. *Heart,* 2009, 95(17): 1436-41.

[45] Bybee, KA; Motiei, A; Syed, IS; Kara, T; Prasad, A; Lennon, RJ; Murphy, JG; Hammill, SC; Rihal, CS; Wright, RS. Electrocardiography cannot reliably differentiate transient left ventricular apical ballooning syndrome from anterior ST-segment elevation myocardial infarction. *J Electrocardiol,* 2007, 40, 38. e1-6.

[46] Abe, Y; Kondo, M; Matsuoka, R; Araki, M; Dohyama, K; Tanio, H. Assessment of clinical features in transient left ventricular apical ballooning. *J Am Coll Cardiol,* 2003, 41, 737-42.

[47] Ogura, R; Hiasa, Y; Takahashi, T. et al. Specific findings of the 12-lead ECG in patients with "takotsubo" cardiomyopathy: comparison with findings of acute anterior myocardial infarction. *Circ J,* 2003, 67, 687-90

[48] Bonnemeier, H; Ortak, J; Bode, F. et al. Modulation of ventricular repolarisation in patients with transient left ventricular apical ballooning: a case control study. *J Cardiovasc Electrophysiol,* 2006, 17(12), 1340-7.

[49] Lemaitre, F; Close, L; Yarol, N. et al. Role of myocardial bridging in the apical localization of stress cardiomyopathy. *Acta cardiol,* 2006, 61(5), 545-50.

[50] Toivonen, L; Helenius, K; Viitasalo, M. Electrocardiographic repolarisation during stress from awakening on alarm call. *J Am Coll Cardiol,* 1997, 30, 774-9.

[51] Diedrich, A; Jordan, J; Shannon, JR; Robertson, D; Biaggioni, I. Modulation of QT interval during autonomic nervous system blockade in humans. *Circulation,* 2002, 106, 2238-43.

[52] Previtali, M; Repetto, A; Panigada, S; Camporotondo, R; Tavazzi, L. Left ventricular apical ballooning syndrome: Prevalence, clinical characteristics and pathogenic mechanisms in a European population. *Int J Cardiol,* 2009, 134, 91-96.

[53] Bahlmann, E; Schneider, C; Krause, K; Hertting, K; Boczor, S; Wollner, T; Voigt, JU; Kuck, KH. Tako-tsubo cardiomyopathy characteristics in long-term follow-up. *Int J Cardiol,* 2008, 124, 32-39.

[54] Merli, ESS; Gori, M; Sutherland, GG. Tako-tsubo cardiomyopathy: new insights into the possible underlying pathophysiology. *Eur J Echocardiogr,* 2006, 7, 53-61.

[55] Donohue, DAC; Sanaei-Ardekani, M; Movahed, MR. Early diagnosis of stress-induced apical ballooning syndrome based on classic echocardiographic findings and correlation with cardiac catheterization. *J Am Soc Echocardiogr,* 2005, 18, 1423.

[56] Elesber, AAPA; Bybee, KA; Valeti, U. et al. Transient cardiac apical ballooning syndrome: prevalence and clinical implications of right ventricular involvement. *J Am Coll Cardiol,* 2006, 7, 1082-3.

[57] Kurisu, S; Inoue, I; Kawagoe, T. et al. Myocardial perfusion and fatty acid metabolism in patients with Takotsubo-like left ventricular dysfunction. *J Am Coll Cardiol,* 2003, 41, 743-8.

[58] Ibanez, B; Navarro, F; Cordoba, M; M-Alberca, P; Farre, J. Tako-tsubo transient left ventricular apical ballooning: is intravascular ultrasound the key to resolve the enigma? *Heart,* 2005, 91, 102-4.

[59] Cattaneo, P; Marchetti, P; Baravelli, M; Rossi, A; Bruno, DV; Anza, C. Could left ventricular apical ballooning represent spontaneous myocardial infraction abortion? *Int J Cardiol,* 2009, 133, e106-108.

[60] Hurst, RT; Askew, JW; Reuss, CS. et al. Transient mid-ventricular ballooning syndrome: a new variant. *J Am Coll Cardiol,* 2006, 48, 579-83.

[61] Yasu, T; Tone, K; Kubo, N; Saito, M. Transient mid-ventricular ballooning cardiomyopathy: a new entity of Takotsubo cardiomyopathy. *Int J Cardiol,* 2006, 110(1), 100-1.

[62] Kurowski, V; Kaiser, A; Von Hof, K. et al. Apical and mid-ventricular transient left ventricular dysfunction syndrome (tako-tsubo cardiomyopathy): frequency, mechanisms and prognosis. *Chest,* 2007, 132(3), 809-16.

[63] Karamitsos, TD; Bull, S; Spyrou, N; Neubauer, B; Selvanayagam, JB. Tako-tsubo cardiomyopathy presenting with features of left ventricular non-compaction. *Int J Cardiol,* 2008, 128(1), e34-6.

[64] Kurisu, S; Inouoe, I; Kawagoe, T. et al. Variant form of tako-tsubo cardiomyopathy. *Int J Cardiol,* 2007, 119(2), e56-8.

[65] Haghi, D; Fleuchter, S; Suselbeck, T; Kaden, JJ; Borggrefe, M; Papavassiliu T. Cardiovascular magnetic resonance findings in typical versus atypical forms of acute apical ballooning syndrome (takotsubo cardiomyopathy). *Int J Cardiol,* 2007, 120, 205-11.

[66] Sharkey, SW; Lesser, JR; Zenovich, AG. et al. Acute and reversible cardiomyopathy provoked by women from the United States. *Circulation,* 2005, 111, 472-9.

[67] Strunk, B; Shaw, RE; Bull, S. et al. High incidence of focal left ventricular wall motion abnormalities and normal coronary arteries in patients with myocardial infarctions presenting to a community hospital. *J Invasive Cardiol,* 2006, 18(8), 376-81.

[68] Akashi, YJ; Nakazawa, K; Sakakibara, M; Miyake, F; Musha, H; Sasaka, K. ^{123}I-MIBG myocardial scintigraphy in patients with "takotsubo" cardiomyopathy. *J Nucl Med,* 2004, 45, 1121-7.

[69] Kurisu, S; Sato, H; Kawagoe, T. et al. Takotsubo-like left ventricular dysfunction with ST-segment elevation: a novel cardiac syndrome mimicking acute myocardial infraction. *Am Heart J,* 2002, 143, 448-55.

[70] Nef, HM; Möllmann, H; Kostin, S; Troidi, C; Voss, S; Weber, M; Dill, T; Rolf, A; Brandt, R; Ham, CW; Elsässer, A. Takotsubo cardiomyopathy: intraindividual structural analysis in the acute phase an after functional recovery. *Eur Heart J,* 2007, 28, 2456-2464.

[71] Karch, SB; Billingham, ME. Myocardial contraction bands revisited. *Hum Pathol,* 1986, 17, 9-13.

[72] Wilkenfeld, C; Cohen, M; Lansman, SL; Courtney, M; Dische, MR; Pertsemlidis, D; Krakoff, LR. Heart transplantation for end-stage cardiomyopathy caused by an occult phaeochromocytoma. *J Heart Lung Transplant,* 1992, 11, 363-36.

[73] Neil-Dwyer, G; Walter, P; Cruickshank, JM; Doshi, B; O'Gorman, P. Effect of propranolol and phentolamine on myocardial necrosis after subarachnoid haemorrhage., *Br Med J,* 1978, 2, 990-2.

[74] Kume, T; Akaaka, T; Kawamoto, T. et al. Assessment of coronary microcirculation in patients with takotsubo-like left ventricular dysfunction. *Circ J,* 2005, 69, 934-9.

[75] Ako, J; Takenaka, K; Uno, K. et al. Reversible left ventricular systolic dysfunction–reversibility of coronary microvascular abnormality. *Jpn Heart J,* 2001, 42, 355-63.

[76] Ellison, GM; Torella, D; Karakikes, I. et al. Acute beta-adrenergic overload produces myocyte damage through calcium leakage from the ryanodine receptor 2 (RYR2) but spares cardiac stem cells. *J Biol Chem,* 2007, 282, 1397-409.

[77] Movahed, A; Reves, WC; Mehta, PM; Gilliand MG; Mozingo, SL; Jolly, SR. Norepinephrine-induced left ventricular dysfunction in anaesthetized and conscious, sedated dogs. *Int J Cardiol,* 1994, 45, 23-33.

[78] Frustaci, A; Loperfido, F; Gentiloni, N; Caldarulo, M; Morgante, E; Russo, MA. Catecholamine-induced cardiomyopathy in multiple endocrine neoplasia: a histological, ultrastructural and biochemical study. *Chest,* 1991, 99, 382-385.

[79] Akashi, YJ; Goldstein, DS; Barbaro, G; Ueyama, T. Takotsubo cardiomyopathy: a new form of acute, reversible heart failure. *Circulation,* 2008, 118, 2754-2762.

[80] Lyon, AR; Rees, PS; Prasad, S; Poole-Wilson, PA; Harding, SE. Stress (Takotsubo) cardiomyopathy: a novel pathophysiological hypothesis to explain catecholamine-induced acute myocardial stunning. *Nat Clin Pract Cardiovasc Med,* 2008, 5, 22-29.

[81] Ueyama, T. Emotional stress-induced Takotsubo cardiomyopathy: animal model and molecular mechanism. *Ann N Y Acad Sci,* 2004, 1018, 437-44.

[82] Villareal, RP; Achari, A; Wilansky, S. et al. Anteroapical stunning and left ventricular outflow tract obstruction. *Mayo Clin Proc,* 2001, 76, 79-83.

[83] Ueyama, T; Kasamatsu, K; Hano, T. et al. Emotional stress induces transient left ventricular hypocontraction in the rat via activation of cardiac adrenoceptors: a possible animal model of 'tako-tsubo' cardiomyopathy. *Circ J,* 2002, 66, 712-3.

[84] Prasad, A; Madhavan, M; Chareonthaitwee, P. Cardiac sympathetic activity in stress-induced (Takotsubo) cardiomyopathy. *Nat Rev Cardiol,* 2009, 6, 430-34.

[85] Sasaki, N; Kinugawa, T; Yamawaki, M; Furuse, Y; Shimoyama, M; Ogino, K; Igawa, O; Hisatome, I; Shigemasa, C. Transient left-ventricular apical ballooning in a patient with bicuspid aortic ale created a left ventricular thrombus leading to acute renal infarction. *Circ J,* 2004, 68, 1081-1083.

[86] Neus Bellera Gotarda, M; Ortiz, JT; Caralt, MT; Pérez-Rodon, J; Mercader, J; Fernández-Gómez, C; Paré, C; Heras, M. Magnetic resonance reveals long-term sequelae of apical ballooning syndrome. *Int J Cardiol,* 2008, In Press.

In: Congestive Heart Failure...   ISBN: 978-1-60876-677-2
Editors: J. E. García et al. pp. 89-109   © 2010 Nova Science Publishers, Inc.

Chapter 4

OXIDATIVE STRESS AND HEART FAILURE: STILL A VIABLE THERAPEUTIC TARGET?

George W. Booz[*]

Department of Pharmacology and Toxicology,
The University of Mississippi School of Medicine,
Jackson, Mississippi, USA

ABSTRACT

The pathogenesis of heart failure is associated with oxidative stress from the generation of reactive oxygen and nitrogen species, which leads to cardiac injury and dysfunction through a variety of means. Yet outcomes of recent interventional studies assessing the utility of anti-oxidants in protecting from cardiovascular disease that can cause heart failure have been disappointing. As discussed here, the ideas behind those studies were perhaps naive and a simple approach of targeting oxidative stress with dietary anti-oxidants is unlikely to be beneficial. The source and nature of the oxidative stress needs to be taken into account in devising therapeutic strategies. Moreover, intracellular redox signaling, which is activated by oxidative stress, plays a key role in cellular protection, as well as tissue repair and regeneration. Consequently, stem

---

[*] Corresponding author: University of Mississippi Medical Center, Department of Pharmacology and Toxicology, 2500 North State Street, Jackson, MS 39216-4505, Tel: (+1) 601-984-4401, Fax: (+1) 601-984-1637, E-mail: gbooz@pharmacology

cell based therapies for heart failure will need to be mindful of the dual nature of oxidative stress to be fully effective.

INTRODUCTION

Oxidative stress describes the situation in which the cell or organ produces reactive oxygen species (ROS), such as superoxide, free radicals, and both organic and inorganic peroxides, in an amount that overwhelms innate detoxification mechanisms [1]. The excess ROS attacks all cellular constituents, not only compromising cellular integrity and function, but inducing intracellular processes that trigger apoptosis or necrosis. Oxidative stress is common to heart failure regardless of the underlying etiology and positively correlates with the degree of dysfunction [1].

Coronary heart disease (CHD) is the leading cause of heart failure. Although all stages of CHD are associated with oxidative events, the role of oxidative damage in its etiology is unsettled [2]. Fueling the controversy are the negative results of recent clinical trials examining anti-oxidant vitamin supplementation as a cardiovascular disease risk modifier, and inconsistent findings on the association of markers of oxidative stress with cardiovascular events. As presented by Bruckdorfer [3], there are many reasons why an anti-oxidant strategy towards treating CHD is unlikely to be successful; however, the take home message is that oxidative stress is an extremely complex phenomenon - not all free radicals are bad, nor are anti-oxidants equally effective. Our understanding of oxidative stress has undergone a maturation over the last several years to where it is now understood as a pathological hyperactivation of normal physiological redox-based signaling events. This knowledge needs to be kept in mind in considering oxidative stress as a therapeutic target in heart failure. Discrete sources of ROS in the failing heart are known and could be selectively targeted either pharmacologically or via molecular means [1]. But a successful anti-oxidant therapeutic approach to heart failure will need also to address the underlying events that led to the excessive ROS production, as well as the fact that the failing heart is an ROS retooled organ.

SOURCES OF OXIDATIVE STRESS IN HEART FAILURE

The major sources of oxidative stress in the failing heart are NADPH oxidases, uncoupled endothelial NO synthase (eNOS), xanthine oxidase, and mitochondria [1]. Although described here individually, intracellular signaling crosstalk is known to occur among them, such that ROS from one source can cause even more ROS generation from another (principally mitochondria). This phenomenon has been termed "ROS-induced ROS release" [4].

The NADPH oxidase (NOX) family of enzymes generates superoxide by transferring electrons from NADPH to molecular oxygen. The superoxide is readily converted to other ROS, including hydrogen peroxide through the enzymatic activity of various superoxide dismutases. NOX exists as a membrane flavocytochrome complex consisting of a catalytic NOX subunit and a smaller $p22^{phox}$ subunit [5,6]. Originally identified in neutrophils, various NOX isoforms were subsequently shown to be fairly ubiquitously expressed and present in all cell types of the heart, including endothelial cells and cardiac myocytes [6]. Cardiac expression and activity of NOX is increased in patients with either ischemic or nonischemic heart failure [6].

Depending upon the isoform involved, the NOX complex may associate with various cytosolic regulatory proteins including Rac1, a member of the ras family of GTPases. Endothelial cells are a rich source of NOX and express both NOX2 and NOX4 [5]. NOX2 is regulated by posttranslational means and is activated by a number of external factors including angiotensin II, certain cytokines, ischemia-reperfusion, and sheer stress. NOX4 does not require any of the known regulatory subunits and appears to be regulated at the transcriptional and post-transcriptional (mRNA stability) levels [6]. Human microvascular endothelial cells may also express NOX5 [5]. Both plasma membrane and intracellular membrane NOX complexes are present in endothelial cells, leading to the idea that subcellular location determines what function the complex has [5]. A substantial body of evidence has implicated NOX activity in both endothelial activation and endothelial dysfunction. Endothelial activation involves changes in endothelial phenotype that contributes to angiogenesis or inflammation, the latter through increased permeability and expression of adhesion molecules and chemokines. NOX is thought to play a major role in endothelial dysfunction, which is impaired endothelium-dependent vasodilator function and is a common feature of heart failure [7]. NOX has been implicated as well in cardiac hypertrophy and interstitial fibrosis [6].

Altogether, NOX would seem to be an excellent therapeutic target in heart failure. While there are currently no drugs that specifically target any of the NOX isoforms, the statins are thought to do so indirectly [8]. The statins are inhibitors of 3-hydroxy-3-methylglutaryl coenzyme A reductase (HMG-CoA reductase), an enzyme involved in the biosynthesis of cholesterol and other isoprenoids. These drugs have proven remarkably effective in primary and secondary prevention of coronary heart disease and myocardial infarction, major causes of heart failure [9,10]. Reducing serum cholesterol largely explains their effectiveness. However, clinical and animal studies have established that their beneficial cardiovascular effects extend beyond serum cholesterol lowering and encompass anti-inflammatory and anti-oxidant actions, leading to improvements in endothelial function [9]. One of several mechanisms thought to contribute to these oft-termed pleiotropic effects is NOX inhibition via reduced activity and expression. The former would result from attenuation of isoprenylation as a consequence of isoprenoid deficiency, thereby precluding activation of the component of NADPH oxidase Rac1 [8]. The question of whether statins offer any benefit once heart failure is established is unsettled [11]. A meta-analysis of 13 studies (11 retrospective and 2 prospective) indicated that statin use among heart failure patients conveys a 26% decreased relative risk of mortality [9]. A subanalysis indicated that statins were equally protective in patients with heart failure of ischemic or nonischemic etiology. In contrast, the findings of 2 large randomized clinical trials were mostly negative for the use of statins in heart failure. In CORONA (Controlled Rosuvastatin Multinational Trial in Heart Failure), 5011 patients with NY Heart Association Class II-IV systolic heart failure of ischemic etiology received 10 mg/ml rosuvastatin daily over a period of approximately 3 years [12]. Although rosuvastatin reduced LDL cholesterol and high sensitivity C-reactive protein (hsCRP) levels, no benefit was seen in terms of strokes, cardiovascular deaths, or heart attacks. Notably, however there was a highly significant reduction in cardiovascular hospitalizations in older patients with advanced systolic heart failure. GISSI-HF (GISSI Heart Failure Trial) assessed the effect of 10 mg/ml rosuvastatin daily in 4594 patients with Class II-IV systolic heart failure of any etiology for nearly 4 years [13]. No benefit was seen in all cause death and hospitalizations for cardiovascular causes. The findings of CORONA and GISSI-HF suggest that statins may be largely beneficial in preventing the progression to coronary artery disease, and ineffective in improving morbidity and mortality once heart failure is established. However, given their excellent safety profile and complications associated with their withdrawal, it has been recommended that statin treatment not be stopped in patients with heart failure [13]. As argued elsewhere, the results of CORONA and GISSI-HF ought not be considered as the last word on the utility of statins in heart failure [14]. For instance, additional clinical studies are needed to evaluate higher dosing levels and, based on CORONA, a composite primary end point focusing on the quality of life.

Others have hypothesized that adjunctive treatment with coenzyme Q_{10} may be required for statins to have benefit in heart failure [15]. Coenzyme Q_{10} is a component of the electron transport chain and potent anti-oxidant found in high concentrations in all cellular membranes, but is particularly rich in the heart. Due to common biosynthetic pathway with cholesterol, statins would be predicted to also lower coenzyme Q_{10} levels; however, there are conflicting reports as to whether or not that is the case [16]. In any event, an early study reported lower levels of coenzyme Q_{10} in endomyocardial biopsy samples and blood from heart failure patients of classes III and IV than those of classes I and II [16]. However, as noted in an expert consensus document published by The American College of Cardiology, the value of coenzyme Q_{10} supplementation in itself in cardiovascular disease is not established [17].

Oxidative stress can lead to a depletion of tetrahydrobiopterin (BH_4), an essential cofactor for the enzymatic activity of eNOS [5,18]. Under this condition, eNOS produces the superoxide anion, a condition referred to as "eNOS uncoupling". A recent animal study highlights the impact of uncoupled eNOS on cardiac function [19]. Treatment of mice with an inhibitor of BH_4 synthetic enzyme GTP cyclohydrolase resulted in cardiac dysfunction, including decreased fractional shortening and increased end-systolic diameter. Cardiac myocytes exhibited a number of contractile defects and abnormal intracellular calcium handling, morphological abnormalities in myocardial filaments and mitochondria, and reduced mitochondrial biogenesis. Notably, all these changes were rescued by cardiac-specific overexpression of the anti-oxidant protein metallothionein.

Xanthine oxidase (XO) catalyzes the oxidation of hypoxanthine to xanthine and xanthine to uric acid, generating superoxide and hydrogen peroxide in the process [20]. The enzyme is reversibly converted to xanthine dehydrogenase by sulfhydryl oxidation, which also catalyzes the oxidation of hypoxanthine to uric acid but with less ROS formation. Both cardiac myocytes and endothelial cells express XO. In the former, XO associates with neuronal nitric oxide synthase (NOS1) in the sarcoplasmic reticulum, which seems to inhibit its activity through S-nitrosylation [20]. In heart failure, XO expression and activity are reported to be increased [21], likely due to elevated levels of angiotensin II and cytokines, ischemia, and the relocation of NOS1 to the sarcolemma. This fact, together with the results of numerous animal studies linking increased XO activity to multiple features of heart failure, such as metabolic and contractile dysfunction, as well as different aspects of cardiac remodeling, fueled expectations that XO inhibition would prove to be a panacea for heart failure [20]. Yet disappointingly, a recent clinical study assessing the efficacy of the potent XO inhibitor oxypurinol in unselected patients with moderate-to-severe heart failure was halted due to lack of clinical improvements [22]. Post-hoc analysis, however, indicated that oxypurinol did benefit patients with elevated serum uric acid levels to a degree that correlated with their reduction in serum uric acid. This finding would suggest that high serum uric acid levels may help identify a subpopulation of heart failure patients likely to benefit from XO inhibition [20]. Three confounding points should be noted: many drugs commonly prescribed for heart failure affect SUA levels, uric acid inhibits xanthine oxidase activity, and uric acid itself is an anti-oxidant [20]. Obviously much more needs to be learned about the role of XO and uric acid in heart failure. Given that XO, along with NADPH oxidase, is an important contributor to vascular oxidative stress, which plays an important role in the progression of vascular endothelial dysfunction, some contribution of XO to heart failure pathogenesies due to coronary heart disease, by far the major cause of heart failure, would seem likely.

Mitochondrial dysfunction of cardiac myocytes is likely the single greatest contributor to the pathogenesis of heart failure, being associated with copious ROS formation, induction of both apoptosis and necrosis, and bioenergetic insufficiency [23,24]. The causes of mitochondrial dysfunction are multifactorial and not totally defined, but are thought to include increased plasma free fatty acids (FFAs), hypoxia, and reactive oxygen species. The latter two are intimately connected in that hypoxia results in increased electron leak from mitochondrial complexes III and II and greater ROS generation. At low levels, mitochondrial ROS plays a role in ischemia preconditioning, a process that protects cardiac myocytes from ischemia-reperfusion injury; however, at higher levels, mitochondrial ROS (together with ROS from other sources) induces further mitochondrial ROS production, resulting in mitochondrial structural damage and ultimately opening of the mitochondrial transition pore (MTP) with dire consequences. But how can this acute catastrophic scenario be reconciled with the chronic insidious nature of heart failure progression? In addition, mitochondria contain several anti-oxidant lines of defense. Recently, a possible enabling condition brought about by reduced calcium loading of mitochondria was proposed that may offer an explanation [25]. Calcium is the signal that couples energy production with demand in cardiac myocytes, since mitochondrial calcium uptake via a uniporter is proportional to cytosolic calcium levels, which in turn reflect the level of contractile activity. Mitochondrial calcium in turn activates certain enzymes of the TCA cycle, thereby increasing NADH production. Besides contributing to ATP production, mitochondrial NADH is critical for maintaining the functionality of many of the anti-oxidant defenses of the mitochondria. Thus, less calcium uptake would be predicted to reduce ATP synthesis and compromise the effectiveness of the ROS scavenging systems of mitochondria. Because of increased cellular sodium in heart failure, calcium uptake by mitochondria may be effectively blunted due to increased calcium efflux from mitochondria via a calcium sodium exchanger [25].

Obviously a drug or molecular therapy that targets (excessive) mitochondrial ROS generation would likely be of benefit in preventing or treating heart failure. A complete discussion of this area is beyond the scope of this review, but 3 investigational drugs or supplements might be mentioned if only to illustrate different possible approaches: PARP inhibitors, SIRT1 activators (e.g., resveratrol), and NHE-1 inhibitors. The nuclear enzyme poly(adenosine diphosphate [ADP]-ribose) polymerase 1 (PARP-1) is involved in DNA repair. Hyperactivation of PARP-1 from oxidative stress–induced DNA strand breakage may result in NAD^+ depletion, preventing synthesis of adenosine triphosphate (ATP) [26]. Additionally, PARP-1 hyperactivation couples to a regulated form of cell death involving intracellular signaling between the nucleus and mitochondria [26]. Hyperactivation of PARP-1 is known to cause mitochondrial depolarization and release of the flavoprotein apoptosis-inducing factor (AIF), which plays a role in maintaining proper functioning of the electron transport chain and oxidative phosphorylation. After being released from mitochondria, AIF translocates to the nucleus where it participates in the condensation and breakdown of chromatin. In animal models, PARP inhibition or genetic deletion offers protection from cardiac ischemia–reperfusion injury, improves cardiac allograft survival, and prevents cardiac hypertrophy and heart failure. SIRT1 is the primary sirtuin or type III histone deacetylase found in the human cell nucleus. Activation of SIRT1, for example by resveratrol, has been shown to protect cells against oxidative stress, in part through the increased expression of anti-oxidant proteins [27]. One such protein is manganese superoxide dismutase (MnSOD), a mitochondrial enzyme that detoxifies superoxde [27]. Finally, the hypertrophied myocardium exhibits enhanced activity of the sarcolemmal Na^+/H^+ exchanger (NHE-1), thought to be from kinase-dependent posttranslational modification downstream of NOX-induced ROS generation [28]. The resultant increased intracellular sodium in turn is thought to stimulate calcium uptake via the Na^+/Ca^{2+} exchanger (NCX), which is postulated to stimulate cardiac hypertrophy via calcineurin, as well as other means, and induce further ROS generation and apoptosis via mitochondrial calcium overload. Consistent with this scheme is recent evidence that NHE-1 inhibitors may be beneficial in preventing heart failure in an animal model [29]. NHE-1 inhibitors also seem to have a direct action on mitochondria to prevent MTP formation and ROS release [30,31].

PHYSIOLOGICAL IMPORTANCE OF REDOX SIGNALING

Although excessive ROS is implicated in cardiac pathologies, there is abundant evidence that at lower levels ROS play an important role in normal cardiac function and repair [5,32]. A full discussion of this subject is beyond the scope of the present work, but several examples are worth noting. First, it was known for many years that coronary blood flow increases linearly with myocardial oxygen consumption, which in turn reflects contractile activity. Endogenous hydrogen peroxide is now thought to be the "metabolic factor" primarily responsible for rapidly regulating the vascular tone of coronary microvessels to match myocardial oxygen supply with demand [33]. Second, γ-glutamyl transpeptidase (GGT) is a ubiquitously expressed plasma membrane enzyme that catalyzes the breakdown of extracellular glutathione, in the process of which superoxide anion is formed [34]. The hydrogen peroxide formed via the dismutation of the superoxide can then initiate intracellular tyrosine kinase signaling that among other consequences is linked to increased gene expression. Recently, evidence was provided that myocardial GGT-induced ROS can be exploited to reverse pathogenic K^+ channel downregulation in the post-MI heart [34]. Finally, it is well established that ROS, most commonly downstream of VEGF stimulation, play a critical role in endothelial cells in varied aspects of angiogenesis, including angiogenesis-related gene expression, as well as endothelial cell migration and proliferation [35]. Just the three examples cited here drive home the point that therapeutic strategies blanketly targeting ROS are likely to be counter-effective to cardiac recovery and repair.

IMPLICATIONS FOR STEM CELL THERAPY

Heart failure, most commonly resulting from myocardial infarction (MI), represents the leading cause of death in developed countries [36-38]. Although strides have been made in recent years in the pharmacological management of heart failure, as well as with the use of devises and surgical interventions, heart failure remains a disease without a cure, short of heart transplantation which is applicable in only a limited number of cases. For that reason, much scientific interest has recently been focused on identifying natural mechanisms for repairing or even regenerating the damaged heart. Foremost among these mechanisms is the use of stem cells. The vast majority of animal studies have shown improvements in both cardiac remodeling and function upon the delivery or mobilization of bone marrow-derived hematopoietic and/or mesenchymal stem cells to the ischemia injured heart [36,37]. Original claims that transdifferentiation of stem cells into cardiac myocytes contributed to those improvements have largely been discredited, however. The current thinking is that stem cell therapy has beneficial effects on the ischemia-assaulted or failing heart because of the plethora of cytokines, chemokines, and growth factors that are secreted by stem cells [38,39]. These paracrine factors are thought to stimulate angiogenesis and cytoprotective mechanisms in heart cells; although some direct contribution of stem/progenitor cells to vasculogenesis and angiogenesis is likely [39,40]. Preliminary human studies assessing the efficacy of stem cells in cardiac repair have also meet with some success; though in general the improvements noted have been more modest than in animal studies. Nonetheless, stem cell delivery has been shown to increase myocardial perfusion and contractile performance in patients with acute MI, coronary artery disease, and chronic ischemia heart failure [38,40]. Evidence from basic research suggests that survivability of stem cells in the injured/stress heart is one limiting factor in the efficacy of stem cell therapy. Manipulations to improve stem cell survivability by enhancing their endogenous protective signaling pathways have resulted in marked improvements in their beneficial actions in the injured heart [36,37].

We use human umbilical cord blood (HUCB) CD34[+] stem cells in our studies. The human umbilical cord offer several advantages over other sources for obtaining stem cells for cardiac cellular therapy, including the following: a relatively higher number of hematopoietic CD34[+] undifferentiated stem/progenitor cells, ready availability without ethical concerns or donor risk, lower risk of graft-versus-host disease (GVHD) owing to naivety of the T-cells, and a higher frequency of rare HLA halotypes [41-43]. In addition, unlike with autologous bone marrow-derived stem cells, disease- or age-related diminution in stem cell potency or viability is not an issue with the use of umbilical cord/placenta stem cell [36,37]. The few disadvantages associated with umbilical cord/placenta stem cell are of little or no concern for cardiovascular indications [42]. The majority of HUCB stem cells are CD34+, representing hematopoietic undifferentiated or progenitor stem cells, and can be easily expanded in culture. In animal studies, HUCB CD34+ cells have been shown to reduce infarct size in the heart, improve cardiac performance, and lead to new blood vessel formation following myocardial infarction [44-47]. Although the evidence indicates that the beneficial effects of HUCB CD34+ cells are principally due the release of paracrine factors with limited differentiation into endothelial cells, two recent studies report that these cells may be capable of transdifferentiating into skeletal and cardiac muscle cells [48,49].

Because of oxidative stress and ROS formation, the ischemic or postischemic myocardium and the hypertrophied or failing heart represent hostile environments for native and recruited cells [50-53]. As is generally the case with stem cells, viability assessments of HUCB CD34+ cells has for the most part been investigated within the framework of apoptosis or less frequently described as necrosis without further clarification. HUCB CD34+ stem cells are reported to undergo apoptosis in response to a variety of manipulations, including long-term culturing or *ex vivo* expansion [54-57], withdrawal or absence of growth factors [58-62], treatment with TNF-α or IFN-γ [61], hypoxia [63], cryopreservation [64-67], and radiation [68,69]. Adult bone marrow-derived human stem and progenitor cells [70-73], and human cord-derived endothelial cell progenitor cells (EPCs) undergo apoptosis in response to oxidative stress [74]. In addition, cryopreservation and radiation are thought to exert a portion of their adverse effects on stem cells through ROS generation [68,75,76].

Accumulating evidence supports a critical role for NOX-mediated redox signaling as the master control system in regulating survivability, growth, and differentiation of human bone marrow-derived and umbilical cord blood hematopoietic stem and progenitor cells [77,78]. The NOX2 and NOX4 isoforms generate superoxide, which is generally converted into H_2O_2 and other ROS. The catalytic activity of the NOX enzymes is enhanced in a positive feedback loop involving ROS, as well as by redox-mediated upregulation of various cytokines. NOX isoforms are also activated by various kinases, for example ERK1/2, and of note are stimulated by environmental conditions, such as hypoxia [79]. Moreover, evidence indicates that some degree of oxidative stress is important for stem cells to produce the appropriate reparative factors. In CD34$^+$ cells, the transcription factor hypoxia-inducible factor-1alpha (HIF-1α) is activated by NOX-generated ROS, leading to increased expression of both vascular endothelial growth factor (VEGF), a potent growth factor for angiogenesis and vasculogenesis, and stromal cell-derived factor-1 (SDF-1), a chemokine that plays an important role in vasculogenesis by recruiting endothelial progenitor cells (EPC) [41,80-82]. However, excessive NOX activity has been implicated in decreased survivability and differentiation of hematopoietic stem/progenitor cells [83-85].

REDOX-SMART DRUG DESIGN FOR HEART FAILURE

Given the pervasive nature of oxidative stress, a strictly anti-oxidant approach in treating heart failure is likely to be palliative at best. Drug strategies to re-engage adversely effected counter measures that also subserve normal cardiac physiological function may prove to be more effective. Two examples of drugs that do just that and which may have utility in heart failure are described here. Metformin is an antihyperglycemic drug that activates AMP-dependent protein kinase (AMPK) and enhances insulin sensitivity. Metanalysis of patients with heart failure and diabetes indicated reduced mortality and hospitalization with metformin [86]. A recent mouse study has provided direct evidence for the effectiveness of metformin in preventing ischemic heart failure. Improvements in cardiac structure and function were attributed to AMPK-mediated activation of eNOS and increased expression of peroxisome proliferator-activated receptor-γ coactivator (PGC)-1α in cardiac myocytes [87]. Besides improving blood flow, NO from enhanced eNOS would be expected to have a number of beneficial opposing actions related to cardiac remodeling [88]. Increased PGC-1α expression was likely the explanation for the noted improvement in mitochondrial respiration and ATP synthesis in this study.

NO- and heme-independent soluble guanylate cyclase (sGC) activators, such as cinaciguat (BAY 58-2667), represent another class of drugs that may prove useful in heart failure [89]. Under normal conditions sGC with its heme moiety is a receptor for NO and is involved in vasodilation and cardioprotection. With oxidative stress, sGC loses its heme and is no longer responsive to NO. However, cinaciguat and other drugs of its class will active oxidized sGC [89,90]. Moreover, they further enhance sGC activity by protecting it from degradation. A recent nonrandomized, uncontrolled, unblinded multicenter phase II study showed that cinaciguat increases cardiac output with potent preload and afterload reducing effects, suggesting that cinaciguat may have use in treating acute decompensated heart failure [91].

CONCLUSION AND PERSPECTIVES

ROS are an integral part of cardiac physiology, which in heart failure become excessive, causing structural and functional damage and contributing to pathological remodeling. Discrete sources of ROS in the failing heart have been identified and shown to act synergistically. Therapeutic approaches that selectively target the sources of ROS and restore their normal level of activity are very much needed. Given the pervasive nature of oxidative stress, as well as the fact that the failing heart is a ROS damaged and retooled heart, a simple anti-oxidant approach to treating heart failure is unlikely to offer much benefit. Combinational strategies to re-engage adversely effected protective measures involved in normal cardiac physiological function are likely to be more effective. Finally, ROS at lower levels play an important role in several aspects of cardiac repair involving cardiac cells, as well as endogenous, recruited, and transplanted stem cells. Finding means to maintain these levels of ROS while reducing excessive ROS production may prove challenging indeed.

ACKNOWLEDGEMENT

This work was supported by a grant from the National Heart, Lung, And Blood Institute (7R01HL088101-02).

REFERENCES

[1]   Seddon, M; Looi, YH; Shah, AM. Oxidative stress and redox signalling in cardiac hypertrophy and heart failure. *Heart.*, 2007, 93, 903-907.

[2]   Mullan, A; Sattar, N. More knocks to the oxidation hypothesis for vascular disease? *Clin Sci (Lond).*, 2009, 116, 41-43.

[3]   Bruckdorfer, KR. Antioxidants and CVD. *Proc Nutr Soc.,* 2008, 67, 214-222.

[4]   Zorov, DB; Filburn, CR; Klotz, LO; Zweier, JL; Sollott, SJ. Reactive oxygen species (ROS)-induced ROS release: a new phenomenon accompanying induction of the mitochondrial permeability transition in cardiac myocytes. *J Exp Med.,* 2000, 192, 1001-1014.

[5]   Sirker, A; Zhang, M; Murdoch, C; Shah, AM. Involvement of Nadph oxidases in cardiac remodelling and heart failure. *Am J Nephrol.,* 2007, 27, 649-660.

[6]   Dworakowski, R; Alom-Ruiz, SP; Shah, AM. NADPH oxidase-derived reactive oxygen species in the regulation of endothelial phenotype. *Pharmacol Rep.,* 2008, 60, 21-28.

[7]   Cave, AC; Brewer, AC; Narayanapanicker, A; Ray, R; Grieve, DJ; Walker, S; Shah, AM. NADPH oxidases in cardiovascular health and disease. *Antioxid Redox Signal.,* 2006, 8, 691-728.

[8]   Förstermann, U. Oxidative stress in vascular disease: causes, defense mechanisms and potential therapies. *Nat Clin Pract Cardiovasc Med.,* 2008, 5, 338-349.

[9]   Ramasubbu, K; Estep, J; White, DL; Deswal, A; Mann, DL. Experimental and clinical basis for the use of statins in patients with ischemic and nonischemic cardiomyopathy. *J Am Coll Cardiol.,* 2008, 51, 415-426.

[10]   Fabbri, G; Maggioni, AP. Cardiovascular risk reduction: What do recent trials with rosuvastatin tell us? *Adv Ther.,* 2009, May, 14. [Epub ahead of print]

[11]   Laufs, U; Custodis, F; Böhm, M. Who does not need a statin: too late in end-stage renal disease or heart failure? *Postgrad Med J.,* 2009, 85, 187-189.

[12]   Kjekshus, J; Apetrei, E; Barrios, V; Böhm, M; Cleland, JG; Cornel, JH; Dunselman, P; Fonseca, C; Goudev, A; Grande, P; Gullestad, L; Hjalmarson, A; Hradec, J; Jánosi, A; Kamenský, G; Komajda, M; Korewicki, J; Kuusi, T; Mach, F; Mareev, V; McMurray, JJ; Ranjith, N; Schaufelberger, M; Vanhaecke, J; van Veldhuisen, DJ; Waagstein, F; Wedel, H; Wikstrand, J; Corona Group. Rosuvastatin in older patients with systolic heart failure. *N Engl J Med.,* 2007, 357, 2248-2261.

[13]   Gissi-HF Investigators; Tavazzi, L; Maggioni, AP; Marchioli, R; Barlera, S; Franzos, MG; Latini, R; Lucci, D; Nicolosi, GL; Porcu, M; Tognoni, G. Effect of rosuvastatin in patients with chronic heart failure

(the GISSI-HF trial): a randomised, double-blind, placebo-controlled trial. *Lancet.*, 2008, 372, 1231-1239.

[14] Serebruany, VL. Controlled rosuvastatin multinational trial in heart failure (the positive negative trial). *Am J Cardiol.*, 2008, 101, 1808-1809.

[15] Okello, E; Jiang, X; Mohamed, S; Zhao, Q; Wang, T. Combined statin/coenzyme Q10 as adjunctive treatment of chronic heart failure. *Med Hypotheses.*, 2009, Apr 29, [Epub ahead of print].

[16] Singh, U; Devaraj, S; Jialal, I. Coenzyme Q10 supplementation and heart failure. *Nutr Rev.*, 2007, 65, 286-293.

[17] Vogel, JH; Bolling, SF; Costello, RB; Guarneri, EM; Krucoff, MW; Longhurst, JC; Olshansky, B; Pelletier, KR; Tracy, CM; Vogel, RA; Vogel, RA; Abrams, J; Anderson, JL; Bates, ER; Brodie, BR; Grines, CL; Danias, PG; Gregoratos, G; Hlatky, MA; Hochman, JS; Kaul, S; Lichtenberg, RC; Lindner, JR; O'Rourke, RA; Pohost, GM; Schofield, RS; Shubrooks, SJ; Tracy, CM; Winters, WL Jr; American College of Cardiology Foundation Task Force on Clinical Expert Consensus Documents (Writing Committee to Develop an Expert Consensus Document on Complementary and Integrative Medicine). Integrating complementary medicine into cardiovascular medicine. A report of the American College of Cardiology Foundation Task Force on Clinical Expert Consensus Documents (Writing Committee to Develop an Expert Consensus Document on Complementary and Integrative Medicine). *J Am Coll Cardiol.*, 2005, 46, 184-221.

[18] Bauersachs, J; Widder, JD. Tetrahydrobiopterin, endothelial nitric oxide synthase, and mitochondrial function in the heart. *Hypertension.*, 2009, 53, 907-908.

[19] Ceylan-Isik, AF; Guo, KK; Carlson, EC; Privratsky, JR; Liao, SJ; Cai, L; Chen, AF; Ren, J. Metallothionein abrogates GTP cyclohydrolase I inhibition-induced cardiac contractile and morphological defects: role of mitochondrial biogenesis. *Hypertension.*, 2009, 53, 1023-1031.

[20] Tziomalos, K; Hare, JM. Role of xanthine oxidoreductase in cardiac nitroso-redox imbalance. *Front Biosci.*, 2009, 14, 237-262.

[21] Cappola, TP; Kass, DA; Nelson, GS; Berger, RD; Rosas, GO; Kobeissi, ZA; Marbán, E; Hare, JM. Allopurinol improves myocardial efficiency in patients with idiopathic dilated cardiomyopathy. *Circulation.*, 2001, 104, 2407-2411.

[22] Hare, JM; Mangal, B; Brown, J; Fisher, C Jr; Freudenberger, R; Colucci, WS; Mann, DL; Liu, P; Givertz, MM; Schwarz, RP; OPT-CHF

Investigators. Impact of oxypurinol in patients with symptomatic heart failure. Results of the OPT-CHF study. *J Am Coll Cardiol.*, 2008, 51, 2301-2309.

[23] Marín-García, J; Goldenthal, MJ. Mitochondrial centrality in heart failure. *Heart Fail Rev.*, 2008, 13, 137-150.

[24] Murray, AJ; Edwards, LM; Clarke, K. Mitochondria and heart failure. *Curr Opin Clin Nutr Metab Care.*, 2007, 10, 704-771.

[25] Liu, T; O'Rourke, B. Regulation of mitochondrial Ca^{2+} and its effects on energetics and redox balance in normal and failing heart. *J Bioenerg Biomembr.*, 2009, 41, 127-132.

[26] Booz, GW. PARP inhibitors and heart failure--translational medicine caught in the act. *Congest Heart Fail.*, 2007, 13, 105-112.

[27] Danz, ED; Skramsted, J; Henry, N; Bennett, JA; Keller, RS. Resveratrol prevents doxorubicin cardiotoxicity through mitochondrial stabilization and the Sirt1 pathway. *Free Radic Biol Med.*, 2009, 46, 1589-1597.

[28] Garciarena, CD; Caldiz, CI; Portiansky, EL; Chiappe de Cingolani, GE; Ennis, IL. Chronic NHE-1 blockade induces an antiapoptotic effect in the hypertrophied heart. *J Appl Physiol.*, 2009, 106, 1325-1331.

[29] Baartscheer, A; Hardziyenka, M; Schumacher, CA; Belterman, CN; van Borren, MM; Verkerk, AO; Coronel, R; Fiolet, JW. Chronic inhibition of the Na^+/H^+-exchanger causes regression of hypertrophy, heart failure, and ionic and electrophysiological remodelling. *Br J Pharmacol.*, 2008, 154, 1266-1275.

[30] Garciarena, CD; Caldiz, CI; Correa, MV; Schinella, GR; Mosca, SM; Chiappe de Cingolani, GE; Cingolani, HE; Ennis, IL. Na^+/H^+ exchanger-1 inhibitors decrease myocardial superoxide production via direct mitochondrial action. *J Appl Physiol.*, 2008, 105, 1706-1713.

[31] Javadov, S; Rajapurohitam, V; Kilić, A; Zeidan, A; Choi, A; Karmazyn, M. Anti-hypertrophic effect of NHE-1 inhibition involves GSK-3β-dependent attenuation of mitochondrial dysfunction. *J Mol Cell Cardiol.*, 2009, 46, 998-1007.

[32] Zima, AV; Blatter, LA. Redox regulation of cardiac calcium channels and transporters. *Cardiovasc Res.*, 2006, 71, 310-321.

[33] Cant, JM Jr; Iyer, VS. Hydrogen peroxide and metabolic coronary flow regulation. *J Am Coll Cardiol.*, 2007, 50, 1279-1281.

[34] Zheng, MQ; Tang, K; Zimmerman, MC; Liu, L; Xie, B; Rozanski, GJ. Role of γ-glutamyl transpeptidase in redox regulation of K^+ channel remodeling in post-myocardial infarction rat hearts. *Am J Physiol Cell Physiol.*, 2009, May 6. [Epub ahead of print].

[35] Ushio-Fukai M. Redox signaling in angiogenesis: role of NADPH oxidase. *Cardiovasc Res.,* 2006, 71, 226-235.

[36] Kurdi, M; Booz, GW. G-CSF-based stem cell therapy for the heart-unresolved issues part A: A: paracrine actions, mobilization, and delivery. *Congest Heart Fail.,* 2007, 13, 221-227.

[37] Kurdi, M; Booz, GW. G-CSF-based stem cell therapy for the heart-unresolved issues part B: stem cells, engraftment, transdifferentiation, and bioengineering. *Congest Heart Fail.,* 2007, 13, 347-351

[38] Leontiadis, E; Manginas, A; Cokkinos, DV. Cardiac repair - fact or fancy? *Heart Fail Rev.,* 2006, 11, 155-170.

[39] Quraishi, A; Losordo, DW. Ischemic tissue repair by autologous bone marrow-derived stem cells: scientific basis and preclinical data. *Handb Exp Pharmacol.,* 2007, 180, 167-179.

[40] Tse, HF; Lau, CP. Therapeutic angiogenesis with bone marrow--derived stem cells. *J Cardiovasc Pharmacol Ther.,* 2007, 12, 89-97.

[41] Goldberg, JL; Laughlin, MJ; Pompili, VJ. Umbilical cord blood stem cells: implications for ardiovascular regenerative medicine. *J Mol Cell Cardiol.,* 2007, 42, 912-920.

[42] Gennery, AR; Cant, AJ. Cord blood stem cell transplantation in primary immune deficiencies. *Curr Opin Allergy Clin Immunol.,* 2007, 7, 528-534.

[43] Goldstein, G; Toren, A; Nagler, A. Transplantation and other uses of human umbilical cord blood and stem cells. *Curr Pharm Des.,* 2007, 13, 1363-1373.

[44] Henning, RJ; Burgos, JD; Ondrovic, L; Sanberg, P; Balis, J; Morgan, MB. Human umbilical cord blood progenitor cells are attracted to infarcted myocardium and significantly reduce myocardial infarction size. *Cell Transplant.,* 2006, 15, 647-658.

[45] Ott, I; Keller, U; Knoedler, M; Götze, KS; Doss, K; Fischer, P; Urlbauer, K; Debus, G; von Bubnoff, N; Rudelius, M; Schömig, A; Peschel, C; Oostendorp, RA. Endothelial-like cells expanded from $CD34^+$ blood cells improve left ventricular function after experimental myocardial infarction. *FASEB J.,* 2005, 19, 992-994.

[46] Botta, R; Gao, E; Stassi, G; Bonci, D; Pelosi, E; Zwas, D, Patti, M; Colonna, L; Baiocchi, M; Coppola, S; Ma, X; Condorelli, G; Peschle, C. Heart infarct in NOD-SCID mice, therapeutic vasculogenesis by transplantation of human $CD34^+$ cells and low dose $CD34^+KDR^+$ cells. *FASEB J.,* 2004, 18, 1392-1394.

[47] Hirata, Y; Sata, M; Motomura, N; Takanashi, M; Suematsu, Y; Ono, M; Takamoto, S. Human umbilical cord blood cells improve cardiac function after myocardial infarction. *Biochem Biophys Res Commun.*, 2005, 327, 609-614.

[48] Pesce, M; Orlandi, A; Iachininoto, MG; Straino, S; Torella, AR; Rizzuti, V; Pompilio, G; Bonanno, G; Scambia, G; Capogrossi, MC. Myoendothelial differentiation of human umbilical cord blood-derived stem cells in ischemic limb tissues. *Circ Res.*, 2003, 93, e51-62.

[49] Condorelli, G; Borello, U; De Angelis, L; Latronico, M; Sirabella, D; Coletta, M; Galli, R,; Balconi, G; Follenzi, A; Frati, G; Cusella De Angelis, MG; Gioglio, L; Amuchastegui, S; Adorini, L; Naldini, L; Vescovi, A; Dejana, E; Cossu, G. Cardiomyocytes induce endothelial cells to trans-differentiate into cardiac muscle: implications for myocardium regeneration. *Proc Natl Acad Sci* U S A., 2001, 98, 10733-10738.

[50] Anilkumar, N; Sirker, A; Shah, AM. Redox sensitive signaling pathways in cardiac remodeling, hypertrophy and failure. *Front Biosci.*, 2009, 14, 3168-187.

[51] Ungvári, Z; Gupte, SA; Recchia, FA; Bátkai, S; Pacher, P. Role of oxidative-nitrosative stress and downstream pathways in various forms of cardiomyopathy and heart failure. *Curr Vasc Pharmacol.*, 2005, 3, 221-229.

[52] Murdoch, CE; Zhang, M; Cave, AC; Shah, AM. NADPH oxidase-dependent redox signalling in cardiac hypertrophy, remodelling and failure. *Cardiovasc Res.*, 2006, 71, 208-215.

[53] Tsutsui, H; Ide, T; Kinugawa, S. Mitochondrial oxidative stress, DNA damage, and heart failure. *Antioxid Redox Signal.*, 2006, 8, 1737-1744.

[54] Hofmeister, CC; Zhang, J; Knight, KL; Le, P; Stiff, PJ. Ex vivo expansion of umbilical cord blood stem cells for transplantation: growing knowledge from the hematopoietic niche. *Bone Marrow Transplant.*, 2007, 39, 11-23.

[55] Astori, G; Larghero, J; Bonfini, T; Giancola, R; Di Riti, M; Rodriguez, L; Rodriguez, M; Mambrini, G; Bigi, L; Lacone, A; Marolleau, JP; Panzani, I; Garcia, J; Querol, S. Ex vivo expansion of umbilical cord blood CD34 cells in a closed system: a multicentric study. *Vox Sang.*, 2006, 90, 183-190.

[56] Tian, H; Huang, S; Gong, F; Tian, L; Chen, Z. Karyotyping, immunophenotyping, and apoptosis analyses on human hematopoietic

precursor cells derived from umbilical cord blood following long-term ex vivo expansion. *Cancer Genet Cytogenet.,* 2005, 157, 33-36.

[57] Seoh, JY; Woo, SY; Im ,SA, Kim, YJ; Park, HY; Lee, S; Lee ,MA; Yoo, ES; Huh, JW; Ryu, KH; Lee, SN; Chung, WS; Seong, CM. Distinct patterns of apoptosis in association with modulation of CD44 induced by thrombopoietin and granulocyte-colony stimulating factor during ex vivo expansion of human cord blood CD34$^+$ cells. *Br J Haematol.,* 1999, 107, 176-85.

[58] Liu, B; Buckley, SM; Lewis, ID; Goldman, AI; Wagner, JE; van der Loo, JC. Homing defect of cultured human hematopoietic cells in the NOD/SCID mouse is mediated by Fas/CD95. *Exp Hematol.,* 2003, 31, 824-832.

[59] Mastino, A; Favalli, C; Camilli, AR; Malerba, C; Grelli, S; Calugi, A. Umbilical cord blood: the role of apoptosis in the control of CD34$^+$ cell counts. *Placenta.,* 2003, 24, 113-115.

[60] Ma, YP; Zou, P; Xiao, J; Huang, SA. Expression of caspase-3 in CD34$^+$ cord blood cells and its significance. *Zhongguo Shi Yan Xue Ye Xue Za Zhi.,* 2002, 10, 387-390.

[61] Ma, Y; Zou, P. Functional expression of CD95/Fas antigen and Bcl-2 on cord blood hematopoietic progenitor cells. *J Huazhong Univ Sci Technolog Med Sci.,* 2002, 22, 24-27.

[62] Wang, LS; Liu, HJ; Xia, ZB; Broxmeyer, HE; Lu, L. Expression and activation of caspase-3/CPP32 in CD34$^+$ cord blood cells is linked to apoptosis after growth factor withdrawal. *Exp Hematol.,* 2000, 28, 907-915.

[63] Dao, MA; Creer, MH; Nolta, JA; Verfaillie, CM. Biology of umbilical cord blood progenitors in bone marrow niches. *Blood.,* 2007, 110, 74-81.

[64] Kurtz, J; Seetharaman, S; Greco, N; Moroff, G. Assessment of cord blood hematopoietic cell parameters before and after cryopreservation. *Transfusion.,* 2007, 47, 1578-1587.

[65] Sparrow, RL; Komodromou, H; Tippett, E; Georgakopoulos, T; Xu, W. Apoptotic lymphocytes and CD34$^+$ cells in cryopreserved cord blood detected by the fluorescent vital dye SYTO 16 and correlation with loss of L-selectin (CD62L) expression. *Bone Marrow Transplant.,* 2006, 38, 61-67.

[66] Greco, NJ; Seetharaman, S; Kurtz, J; Lee, WR; Moroff, G. Evaluation of the reactivity of apoptosis markers before and after cryopreservation in cord blood CD34$^+$ cells. *Stem Cells Dev.,* 2006, 15, 124-135.

[67] Shim, JS; Cho, B; Kim, M; Park, GS; Shin, JC; Hwang, HK; Kim, TG; Oh, IH. Early apoptosis in CD34$^+$ cells as a potential heterogeneity in quality of cryopreserved umbilical cord blood. *Br J Haematol.*, 2006, 135, 210-213.

[68] Hayashi, T; Hayashi, I; Shinohara, T; Morishita, Y; Nagamura, H; Kusunoki, Y; Kyoizumi, S; Seyama, T; Nakachi, K. Radiation-induced apoptosis of stem/progenitor cells in human umbilical cord blood is associated with alterations in reactive oxygen and intracellular pH. *Mutat Res.*, 2004, 556, 83-91.

[69] Kashiwakura, I; Inanami, O; Takahashi, K; Takahashi, TA; Kuwabara, M; Takagi, Y. Protective effects of thrombopoietin and stem cell factor on X-irradiated CD34$^+$ megakaryocytic progenitor cells from human placental and umbilical cord blood. *Radiat Res.*, 2003, 160, 210-216.

[70] Zhang, X; Sejas, DP; Qiu, Y; Williams, DA; Pang, Q. Inflammatory ROS promote and cooperate with the Fanconi anemia mutation for hematopoietic senescence. *J Cell Sci.*, 2007, 120, 1572-1583.

[71] Tothova, Z; Kollipara, R; Huntly, BJ; Lee, BH; Castrillon, DH; Cullen, DE; McDowell, EP; Lazo-Kallanian, S; Williams, IR; Sears, C; Armstrong, SA; Passegué, E; DePinho, RA; Gilliland, DG. FoxOs are critical mediators of hematopoietic stem cell resistance to physiologic oxidative stress. *Cell.*, 2007, 128, 325-339.

[72] Sasnoor, LM; Kale, VP; Limaye, LS. Prevention of apoptosis as a possible mechanism behind improved cryoprotection of hematopoietic cells by catalase and trehalose. *Transplantation.*, 2005, 80, 1251-1260.

[73] Zhang, X; Li, J; Sejas, DP; Pang, Q. The ATM/p53/p21 pathway influences cell fate decision between apoptosis and senescence in reoxygenated hematopoietic progenitor cells. *J Biol Chem.*, 2005, 280, 19635-19640.

[74] Ingram, DA; Krier, TR; Mead, LE; McGuire, C; Prater, DN; Bhavsar, J; Saadatzadeh, MR; Bijangi-Vishehsaraei, K; Li, F; Yoder, MC; Haneline, LS. Clonogenic endothelial progenitor cells are sensitive to oxidative stress. *Stem Cells.*, 2007, 25, 297-304.

[75] Yard, B; Beck, G; Schnuelle, P; Braun, C; Schaub, M; Bechtler M; Göttmann, U; Xiao, Y; Breedijk, A; Wandschneider, S; Lösel, R; Sponer, G; Wehling, M; van der Woude, FJ. Prevention of cold-preservation injury of cultured endothelial cells by catecholamines and related compounds. *Am J Transplant.*, 2004, 4, 22-30.

[76] Sasnoor, LM; Kale, VP; Limaye, LS. Prevention of apoptosis as a possible mechanism behind improved cryoprotection of hematopoietic cells by catalase and trehalose. *Transplantation.*, 2005, 80, 1251-1260.

[77] Piccoli, C; D'Aprile, A; Ripoli, M; Scrima, R; Boffoli, D; Tabilio, A; Capitanio, N. The hypoxia-inducible factor is stabilized in circulating hematopoietic stem cells under normoxic conditions. *FEBS Lett.*, 2007, 581, 3111-3119.

[78] Piccoli, C; D'Aprile, A; Ripoli, M; Scrima, R; Lecce, L; Boffoli, D; Tabilio, A; Capitanio, N. Bone-marrow derived hematopoietic stem/progenitor cells express multiple isoforms of NADPH oxidase and produce constitutively reactive oxygen species. *Biochem Biophys Res Commun.*, 2007, 353, 965-972.

[79] Abdallah, Y; Gligorievski, D; Kasseckert, SA; Dieterich, L; Schäfer, M; Kuhlmann, CR; Noll, T; Sauer, H; Piper, HM; Schäfer, C. The role of poly(ADP-ribose) polymerase (PARP) in the autonomous proliferative response of endothelial cells to hypoxia. *Cardiovasc Res.* 2007;73, 568-574.

[80] Milovanova, TN; Bhopale, VM; Sorokina, EM; Moore, JS; Hunt, TK; Hauer-Jensen, M; Velazquez, OC; Thom, SR. Hyperbaric oxygen stimulates vasculogenic stem cell growth and differentiation in vivo. *J Appl Physiol.*, 2009, 106, 711-728.

[81] Milovanova, TN; Bhopale, VM; Sorokina, EM; Moore, JS; Hun,t TK; Hauer-Jensen, M; Velazquez, OC; Thom, SR. Lactate stimulates vasculogenic stem cells via the thioredoxin system and engages an autocrine activation loop involving hypoxia-inducible factor 1. *Mol Cell Biol.*, 2008, 28, 6248-6261.

[82] Kietzmann, T; Görlach, A. Reactive oxygen species in the control of hypoxia-inducible factor-mediated gene expression. *Semin Cell Dev Biol.*, 2005, 16, 474-486.

[83] Piccoli, C; Ria, R, Scrima, R; Cela, O; D'Aprile, A; Boffoli, D; Falzetti, F; , A; Capitanio, N. Characterization of mitochondrial and extra-mitochondrial oxygen consuming reactions in human hematopoietic stem cells. Novel evidence of the occurrence of NAD(P)H oxidase activity. *J Biol Chem.*, 2005, 280, 26467-26476.

[84] Thum, T; Fraccarollo, D; Thum, S; Schultheiss, M; Daiber, A; Wenzel, P; Munzel, T; Ertl, G; Bauersachs, J. Differential effects of organic nitrates on endothelial progenitor cells are determined by oxidative stress. *Arterioscler Thromb Vasc Biol.*, 2007, 27, 748-754.

[85] Werner, C; Kamani, CH; Gensch, C; Böhm, M; Laufs, U. The peroxisome proliferator-activated receptor-γ agonist pioglitazone increases number and function of endothelial progenitor cells in patients with coronary artery disease and normal glucose tolerance. *Diabetes.*, 2007, 56, 2609-2615.

[86] Eurich, DT; McAlister, FA; Blackburn, DF; Majumdar, SR; Tsuyuki, RT; Varney, J; Johnson, JA. Benefits and harms of antidiabetic agents in patients with diabetes and heart failure: systematic review. *BMJ.*, 2007, 335, 497.

[87] Gundewar, S; Calvert, JW; Jha, S; Toedt-Pingel, I; Ji, SY; Nunez, D, Ramachandran, A; Anaya-Cisneros, M; Tian, R; Lefer, DJ. Activation of AMP-activated protein kinase by metformin improves left ventricular function and survival in heart failure. *Circ Res.*, 2009, 104, 403-411.

[88] Booz, GW. Putting the brakes on cardiac hypertrophy: exploiting the NO-cGMP counter-regulatory system. *Hypertension.*, 2005, 45, 341-346.

[89] Schmidt, HH; Schmidt, PM; Stasch, JP. NO- and haem-independent soluble guanylate cyclase activators. *Handb Exp Pharmacol.*, 2009, 309-339.

[90] Boerrigter, G; Burnett, JC Jr. Soluble guanylate cyclase: not a dull enzyme. *Circulation.*, 2009, 119, 2752-2754.

[91] Lapp, H; Mitrovic, V; Franz, N; Heuer, H; Buerke, M; Wolfertz, J; Mueck, W; Unger, S; Wensing, G; Frey, R. Cinaciguat (BAY 58-2667) improves cardiopulmonary hemodynamics in patients with acute decompensated heart failure. *Circulation.*, 2009, 119, 2781-2788.

In: Congestive Heart Failure...   ISBN: 978-1-60876-677-2
Editors: J. E. García et al. pp. 111-127 © 2010 Nova Science Publishers, Inc.

Chapter 5

SIMULATING CALCINEURIN-CENTERED CALCIUM SIGNALING NETWORK IN CARDIAC MYOCYTES

Jiangjun Cui[1]*, Jaap A. Kaandorp[2], Peter M. A. Sloot[2] and P. S. Thiagarajan[1]

[1]Department of Computer Science, National University of Singapore, Blk COM1, 13 Computing Drive, Singapore 117417
[2]Section Computational Science, University of Amsterdam, Science Park 107, 1098 XG Amsterdam, the Netherlands

ABSTRACT

Calcium ion has been found to play critical roles regulating both the beating and the growth of the heart. Mathematical modeling and computational simulations are required for understanding the complex dynamics arising from the calcium signaling networks controlling the heart growth, which is critical for devising therapeutic drugs for the treatment of pathologic hypertrophy and heart failure. In this paper, we will report our newest results of simulating the relevant calcineurin-centered calcium signaling pathways under the hypertrophic stimulus of pressure overload. We will show how the dual roles of RCAN protein in cardiac hypertrophy under different hypertrophic stimuli can be explained

---

* Corresponding author: {cuijj,thiagu}@comp.nus.edu.sg

by the complex interactions of multiple signaling pathways and indicate how this particular example can help us understand the mystery of specificity encoding in calcium signaling networks. We will also discuss how to push forward the realistic modeling of calcium signaling network in mammalian hearts and how it can benefit from the corresponding calcium signaling research in simpler organisms such as yeast.

Keywords: calcium homeostasis, calcium signaling, cardiac myocytes, cardiac hypertrophy, calcineurin

1. INTRODUCTION

In eukaryotic cells, Ca^{2+} functions as a highly versatile intracellular messenger regulating a myriad of cellular processes such as proliferation, muscle contraction, neurotransmitter release, programmed cell death, etc [5-7, 30,33]. Calcium homeostasis systems are highly regulated metabolic pathways to maintain Ca^{2+} at optimal concentration ranges in its cytosol and other organelles. Normally a biological cell maintains an extremely high gradient of Ca^{2+} concentration across the cell membranes through the functioning of its calcium homeostasis system involving coordination between ion uptake, distribution, storage and efflux. Extracellular stimuli cause the change of the opening probability of various calcium transport proteins (mostly channels) on the membranes and results in sudden calcium influx into the cytosol due to the extremely high gradient. Calcium signaling depends on the increased levels of cytosolic Ca^{2+} concentrations derived either from sources outside the cell or within the organelles such as ER/SR (in mammalian and plant cells. ER: endoplasmic reticulum; SR: sarcoplasmic reticulum) and/or the vacuole (in plant and yeast cells) to activate the effector proteins to exert a cellular response [6,7,11,13,14].

The novelty of calcium signaling was firstly demonstrated by a "mistaken" experiment conducted by British clinician and pharmacologist Sidney Ringer (1836-1910) who used

London tap water (instead of distilled water) containing calcium at nearly the same concentration as the blood to make a saline medium for suspending isolated rat hearts [9].

The beating of the hearts became progressively weaker and eventually stopped when the tap water was replaced by distilled water. Since then, the mysterious fog covering the iceberg of calcium signaling was gradually unveiled and now calcium is regarded as the most versatile signaling molecule regulating a myriad of important processes both inside and outside the cells [5-7,9].

Although the role of calcium ion as a central regulator in heart beating has been established by Sidney Ringer as early as 1880s, the critical role of calcium ion in the regulation of heart growth has just recently been recognized. For example, the complex calcium-calcineurin-RCAN-NFAT signaling network shown in Figure 1 describes the experimentally found calcineurin-dependent calcium signaling pathways controlling the heart growth under the hypertrophic stimuli (stress) such as pressure overload (PO) and active calcineurin (CaN*) overexpression [12]. This network is a part of the group of signal-transduction pathways which have recently been characterized to be implicated in the regulation of cardiac hypertrophy [22]. The activation of different pathways appears to be specific for the stimulus [38].

As shown in the left-up corner of Figure 1, calmodulin (CaM), a universal calcium sensor protein, senses the raised level of cytosolic Ca^{2+} incurred by stress. Ca^{2+}-bound CaM binds to a protein phosphatase called calcineurin (CaN) to activate it. The regulator of calcineurin (RCAN) can bind CaN* (i.e., active CaN) to form Complex1 [42,43]. CaN* can dephosphorylate phospho-NFAT ($NFAT^P$) and promote its translocation from cytoplasm into the nucleus. The phosphorylation of NFAT into $NFAT^P$ is mediated by kinase GSK3β. A protein called 14-3-3 can bind $NFAT^P$ to form Complex3 [27]. Both GSK3β and CaN* are shuttled between the cytosol and the nucleus, where they mediate the phosphorylation of NFAT and dephosphorylation of $NFAT^P$, respectively [20]. NFAT in the cytosol is imported into the nucleus to initiate the transcription of the hypertrophic genes and the gene encoding RCAN (more precisely, RCAN1, a form of RCAN). $NFAT^P$ in the nucleus is exported into the cytosol. A kinase called BMK1 is only activated by particular stress such as PO (see the right-up corner of Figure 1, [40]) and it is the priming kinase responsible for phosphorylating RCAN into $RCAN^P$, whose further phosphorylation into $RCAN^{PP}$ is mediated by GSK3β. CaN* is responsible for mediating the dephosphorylation of $RCAN^{PP}$ into $RCAN^P$. $RCAN^{PP}$ can bind protein 14-3-3 to form Complex2 [1].

The role of RCAN in cardiac hypertrophy has been experimentally shown to be paradoxical. RCAN1 seems to facilitate calcineurin signaling under certain stress conditions such as PO and isoproterenol (ISO) infusion whereas it suppresses calcineurin signaling under some other stress conditions such as CaN* overexpression (see Figure 3a).

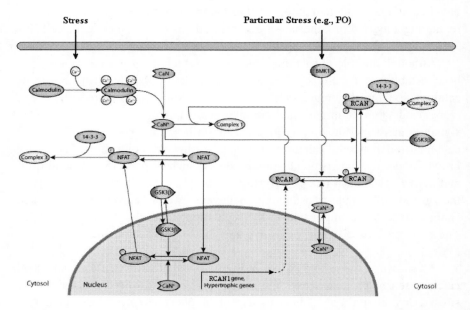

Figure 1. A schematic graph depicting the Ca2+-calcineurin-RCAN-NFAT signaling network in cardiac myocytes (this figure is modified after the CellML version of the model developed by Cui & Kaandorp, see *http://www.cellml.org/models*) [12]. Abbreviations are as follows: calmodulin (CaM); calcineurin (CaN); active calcineurin (CaN*); nuclear factor of activated T-cells (NFAT); phosphorylated NFAT(NFAT^P); regulator of calcineurin (RCAN, also named as calcipressin, Down syndrome critical region (DSCR) and modulatory calcineurin-interacting protein (MCIP)); phosphorylated RCAN on serine 112 (RCAN^P); phosphorylated RCAN on both serine 112 and serine 108 (RCAN^{PP}); big mitogen-activated protein kinase 1 (BMK1); glycogen synthase 3β (GSK3β); the complex formed by RCAN and calcineurin (Complex1); the complex formed by RCAN^{PP} and 14-3-3 (Complex2); the complex formed by NFAT^P and 14-3-3 (Complex3); pressure overload (PO); hypertrophic stimuli (stress).

2. METHODS & SIMULATION RESULTS

To simulate the dynamics of the complex Ca^{2+}-calcineurin signaling network shown in Figure 1, we decomposed the network into 17 reactions in addition to a transcriptional control process of RCAN by nuclear NFAT and constructed a mathematical model composed of 28 ordinary differential equations which were automatically generated using Cellerator software (the detailed equations and initial conditions are described in the Appendix. For details of the relevant reactions and the values of parameters, please see [12]). A selected steady state[1] was used for simulating the normally growing heart cells. The stimulus of PO was simulated by simultaneously setting the simulated cytosolic calcium concentration to a higher level and increasing the initial value of active BMK1 concentration because PO increases the cytosolic calcium level and activates BMK1 [40]. The stimulus of CaN* overexpression[2] was simulated in a similar way (see Appendix) [12].

In Figure 2, critical transient curves in the case of PO for simulated wildtype (i.e., RCAN$^{+/+}$) cells are shown. From Figure 2a, we can see that due to pressure overload, cytosolic CaN* rises (in less than 1 hour) to a high peak of 0.33 μM, drops to around 0.3 μM (see the inset) and then very gradually declines (it eventually rests at a level of 0.105 μM). From Figure 2b, we can see that the concentration of RCAN^P and RCAN^{PP} gradually increases from 0 μM to 2.9 μM and 4.3 μM in 60 weeks, respectively, whereas the concentration of RCAN remains almost 0 in the whole process. From Figure 2c, we can see that the concentration of Complex2 gradually increases from 0.283 μM to a resting level of 0.96 μM whereas the concentration of Complex1 increases from almost 0 to around 0.29 μM. The concentration of 14-3-3 decreases from 0.71 μM to 0.044 μM. From Figure 2d, we can see that the concentration of nuclear NFAT rises from 4.99 nM to a resting value of 7.2 nM whereas cytosolic NFAT^P (i.e., $NFATpc(t)$) firstly decreases quickly from 4.9 nM to around 3 nM and then gradually recovers to a new resting level of 8.9 nM. The concentration of Complex3 decreases from 14 nM to a final resting level of 1.6 nM. Similar as Shin et al.[3] (2006) did in their paper, we can use the integral of nuclear NFAT concentration (i.e., $\int_0^t NFATn(\delta)d\delta$) as a measure for the extent of hypertrophic response. The simulated hypertrophic responses for wild type (i.e., RCAN$^{+/+}$) and RCAN mutant (i.e., RCAN$^{-/-}$) mice under the stimuli of CaN* overexpression and PO are depicted as a function of time in Figure 3b.

---

[1] In this model, the cytosolic calcium level is regarded as a constant because we are only simulating calcineurin-dependent calcium signaling systems and calcineurin is well-known for its specific responsiveness to sustained, low frequency calcium signals (see Shin et al., 2006 for the origin of this idea) [12,37].

[2] CaN* expression was experimentally realized by overexpressing a constitutively active calcineurin in transgenic mouse (TG) hearts [43].

[3] Please note that Cui and Kaandorp, 2008 is a much–extended version of the model built by Shin et al., 2006 [12,37].

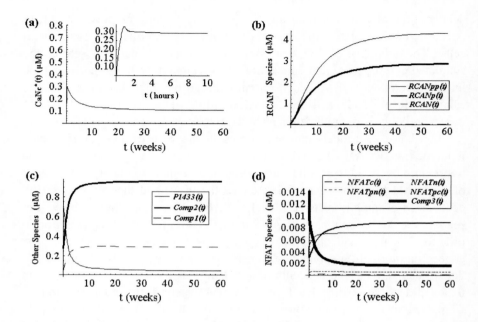

Figure 2. Simulated transient curves for normal animals under the stimulus of pressure overload. (a) Simulated $CaNc^*(t)$ (i.e., cytosolic CaN*) as a function of t. The inset figure in the right-up corner shows the detailed change of $CaNc^*(t)$ during the first 50 minutes. (b) Simulated concentration of RCAN species as a function of t. Thin solid line: $RCANpp(t)$; thick solid line: $RCANp(t)$; dashed line: $RCAN(t)$. Please note that the dashed line coincides with the t axis. (c) Simulated concentration of some other species as a function of t. Thin solid line: $P1433(t)$; thick solid line: $Comp2(t)$; dashed line: $Comp1(t)$. (d) Simulated NFAT species concentration as a function of t. Thin solid line: $NFATn(t)$; thick solid line: $NFATpc(t)$; extremely thick solid line: $Comp3(t)$; sparsely dashed line (bottom): $NFATc(t)$; densely dashed line: $NFATpn(t)$. Abbreviations and synonyms used are as follows: RCAN^P (RCANp); RCAN^{PP} (RCANpp); NFAT^P (NFATp); cytosolic NFAT (NFATc); cytosolic NFATp (NFATpc); cytosolic inactive CaN (CaNc); cytosolic CaN* (CaNc*); cytosolic GSK3β (GSK3βc); nuclear NFAT (NFATn); nuclear NFATp (NFATpn); nuclear CaN* (CaNn*); nuclear GSK3β (GSK3βn); 14-3-3 protein (P1433); Ca^{2+}-bound CaM (CaMCa); Complex1 (Comp1); Complex2 (Comp2); Complex3 (Comp3).

3. DISCUSSIONS

The increase of Complex2 shown in Figure 2c means the accelerated formation of Complex2 which should consume more $RCAN^{PP}$ (see Figure 1). However, from Figure 2b, we can see that the concentration of $RCAN^{PP}$ is actually increasing. This can only be explained by that the activation of BMK1 catalyzes the conversion of RCAN to $RCAN^{P}$ and then to $RCAN^{PP}$ and the resultant abundance of $RCAN^{PP}$ promotes the formation of Complex2, which also causes the concentration decrease of 14-3-3 as seen in Figure 2c. The depletion of 14-3-3 promotes the dissociation of Complex3 (see Figure 2d, the extremely thick line) which releases more cytosolic $NFAT^{P}$. By comparison of these simulation results with those for $RCAN^{-/-}$ cell shown in Figure 3c-d, we can see that in mutant cell, the concentration of Complex3 decreases much more rapidly to a much higher resting level (please compare the extremely thick line in Figure 2d with that in Figure 3d) which means that the inhibitory effect of 14-3-3 on hypertrophic response under PO becomes more severe due to the lack of RCAN. In another word, in $RCAN^{+/+}$ cell, PO activates BMK1 to promote the formation of phosphorylated RCAN (i.e., $RCAN^{PP}$) which associates with 14-3-3 to relieve its inhibitory effect on hypertrophic response. Conversely, in the case of CaN* overexpression (for relevant simulation results, please see [12]), the abundance of active calcineruin promotes $RCAN^{PP} \rightarrow RCAN^{P} \rightarrow RCAN$ which associates with CaN* to inhibit its activity. Moreover, newly expressed RCAN also makes significant contribution to this inhibition.

From Figure 3b, we can see that after a typical period (8 weeks) of growth [43], the end point of simulated hypertrophic response (the thin solid line) for $RCAN^{+/+}$ CaN* TG mice is much lower than that for $RCAN^{-/-}$ CaN* TG mice (the thick solid line) whereas the end point of simulated hypertrophic response (the sparsely dashed line) for $RCAN^{+/+}$ mice under the PO stimulus is higher than that of $RCAN^{-/-}$ mice (the densely dashed line). These simulation results are in accordance with the seemingly dual role of RCAN (see Figure 2a) in cardiac hypertrophy which has been found experimentally [43].

As mentioned at the very beginning, Ca^{2+} is the most ubiquitous and versatile intracellular messenger. Therefore, it is quite natural that people are very interested in the specificity encoding in calcium signaling networks, i.e., how does Ca^{2+} performs its function with strict specificity to link different stimuli to their corresponding cellular response? Several hypotheses have been proposed to explain this mysterious and intriguing open question. The most

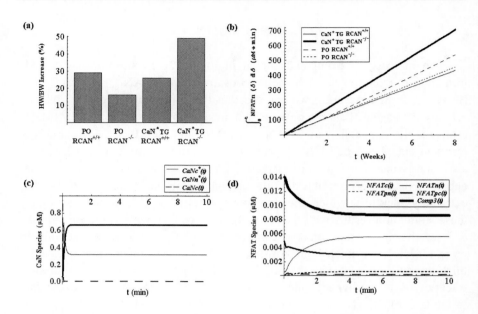

Figure 3. Comparison of experimentally reported and simulated hypertrophic response. (a) RCAN1 seems to facilitate or suppress cardiac CaN signaling depending on the nature of the stress. In the case of CaN* overexpression (expressed from a muscle-specific transgene), the knockout of RCAN1 gene exacerbated the hypertrophic response (please compare the height of the fourth bar with that of the third bar). Paradoxically, however, cardiac hypertrophy in response to PO was blunted in normal RCAN$^{-/-}$ mice (please compare the height of the first two bars) [43]. (b) The simulated hypertrophic response for wildtype (i.e., RCAN$^{+/+}$) and RCAN mutant (i.e., RCAN$^{-/-}$) mice under the stimuli of CaN* overexpression and PO.

dominant hypothesis is called "calcium signature hypothesis", which assumes that the temporal and spatial nature and the amplitude of the cytosolic calcium concentration change constitutes a signature encoding the calcium signals, which are later decoded by the downstream effector proteins [5,18,32,41]. Many experimental evidences have been found supporting this well-known hypothesis [2,16,26,29]. A contrary theory called "chemical switch hypothesis" was proposed by Scrase-Field et al. (2003) arguing that calcium ion may work as a chemical switch and specificity in calcium signaling networks can be encoded by components other than calcium [35]. Our work presented here shows a good example of that specificity can be encoded in the complex cross-interaction of multiple signaling pathways, thus supporting the "chemical switch hypothesis" (Please note that both the calcium-calcineruin-

NFAT pathway and the BMK1/ERK5[4] signaling pathway are activated in the case of PO induced cardiac hypertrophy whereas the BMK1/ERK5 signaling pathway is not activated in the case of CaN* overexpression).

The calcium homeostasis/signaling process in mammalian cardiac myocytes exhibits extreme complexity, of which Figure 1 describes only a part of the whole picture [14,22]. Besides calcineurin-dependent pathways, other calcium signaling pathways such as CAMK (calmodulin-dependent kinase)-dependent pathways have been characterized to be involved in the regulation of cardiac hypertrophy [22]. Moreover, apart from the calcium signaling pathways regulating the long term cardiac growth process, mammalian cardiac mycocytes has a set of signaling toolkits composed of channels (e.g., L-Type Ca^{2+} Channel (LTCC), ryanodine receptor (RyR)), pumps (e.g., sarcoplasmic reticulum Ca^{2+}-ATPase (SERCA)), exchangers and other relevant components to regulate the short-term cardiac excitation-contraction process [3,8]. This great number of involved factors, in addition to the extremely sophisticated regulations, the built-in coupling with other ion (e.g., Na^+ and K^+) homeostasis and the very important spatial and stochastic effects makes the accurate approximate of cardiac calcium signaling process to be a formidable and daunting task [14].

Although many computational models about calcium homeostasis/signaling networks in cardiac myocytes have been published in past decades, they are all quite preliminary works and far from being accurate approximation [12,19,31,36,39]. In order to push forward the realistic modeling of the calcium signaling network in mammalian hearts, from experimental point of view, we need to develop more advanced imaging techniques to monitor the spatial and temporal changes of calcium concentration in various organelles of cardiac myocytes [34,44]; from modeling point of view, we need to:

(i)   identify the missing components of calcium signaling networks and determining the relevant rate constants;
(ii) develop effective computational methods to approximate the calcium-dependent reaction-diffusion processes in cardiac myocytes of complex geometry [10];
(iii) develop novel computational methods (e.g., molecular dynamics method) to capture the stochastic and microdomain signaling events which have been proven to play important role [4,8].

---

[4] ERK5 is a synonym of BMK1 [21].

None of the above three sub-tasks are easy.

4. CONCLUSION

To summarize, our simulation results show that RCAN is essentially an inhibitor of calcineurin and the seemingly facilitating role of RCAN on calcineurin signaling under the stimulus of PO can be explained by the accelerated formation of phosphorylated RCAN (i.e., $RCAN^{PP}$) which associates with 14-3-3 to relieve its inhibitory effect on cardiac hypertrophy. To achieve realistic understanding of calcium homeostasis/signaling process in cardiac myocytes is a typical systems biology problem imposing great experimental and computational challenges and it still needs a long way to go [17].

Very recently, we have shown that many components and quite a few mechanisms of yeast calcium homeostasis/signaling system are well conserved in mammalian cardiac myocytes [14]. For example, RCAN1 has a functional counterpart protein named as Rcn1 in yeast system whose regulation on calcineurin activity also exhibits similarly paradoxical role while the functional counterpart of GSK3β in yeast calcium system is Mck1 [23,24]. Recent experimental evidence has shown that Mck1-dependent phosphorylation targets Rcn1 for degradation through the SCF^{Cdc4} and relieves the inhibition of calcineurin [25]. Thus it would be interesting to examine whether similar mechanism exists in mammalian cardiac myocytes.

Since yeast is a unicellular organism that affords powerful genetic and genomic tools, it is much easier to push forward the realistic approximation of yeast calcium homeostasis/signaling system, whose understanding can be a shortcut to help identify the missing components and understand the regulatory mechanisms in the mammalian cardiac calcium signaling system and treat relevant human diseases such as pathological cardiac hypertrophy and heart failure [12,14,30].

ACKNOWLEDGEMENTS

We would like to thank Prof. Kyle W. Cunningham (Johns Hopkins University, USA) for his suggestion of the topic and stimulating discussions. We thank Dr. Catherine M. Lloyd for translating the relevant model (Cui &

Kaandorp 2008a) into CellML code (http://www.cellml.org/models 2008_version02) and include it into the CellML Model Repository [28]. J. Cui was firstly funded by the Dutch Science

Foundation on the project ``Mesoscale simulation paradigms in the silicon cell'', later supported by two grants from the EC on MORPHEX (NEST Contract No. 043322) and QosCos projects, and recently by NUS grant (R-252-000-350-112) for the project "Decomposition and composition of large signaling pathway models with emphasis on parameter estimation".

REFERENCES

[1]   Abbasi, S., Lee, J. D., Su, B., Chen, X., Alcon, J. L., Yang, J., Kellems, R. E. & Xia, Y. (2006). Protein kinase-mediated regulation of calcineurin through the phosphorylation of modulatory calcineurin-interacting protein 1. *J Biol Chem*, *281*, 7717-7726.

[2]   Allen, G. J., Chu, S. P., Schumacher, K., Shimazaki, C. T., Vafeados, D., Kemper, A., Hawke, S. D., Tallman, G., Tsien, R. Y., Harper, J. F., Chory, J. & Schroeder, J. I. (2000). Alteration of stimulus-specific guard cell calcium oscillations and stomatal closing in *Arabidopsis* det3 mutant. *Science*, *289*, 2338-2342.

[3]   Barry, W. H. & Bridge, J. H. (1993). Intracellular calcium homeostasis in cardiac myocytes. *Circulation*, *87*, 1806-1815.

[4]   Beckstein, O., Biggin, P. C., Bond, P., Bright, J. N., Domene, C., Grottesi, A., Holyoake, J. & Sansom, M. S. P. (2003). Ion channel gating: insights via molecular simulations. *FEBS Lett*, *555*, 85-90.

[5]   Berridge, M. J., Bootman, M. D. & Lipp, P. (1998). Calcium - a life and death signal. *Nature*, *395*, 645-648.

[6]   Berridge, M. J., Bootman, M. D. & Roderick, H. L. (2003). Calcium signaling: dynamics, homeostasis and remodeling. *Nat Rev Mol Cell Biol*, *4*, 517-529.

[7]   Berridge, M. J., Lipp, P. & Bootman, M. D. (2000). The versatility and universality of calcium signaling. *Nat Rev Mol Cell Biol*, *1*, 11-21.

[8]   Bers, D. M. (2002). Cardiac excitation–contraction coupling. *Nature*, *415*, 198-205.

[9]   Carafoli, E. (2000). Calcium signaling: a tale for all seasons. *Proc Natl Acad Sci USA*, *99*, 1115-1122.

[10] Cheng, H., Lederer, M. R., Lederer, W. J. & Cannell, M. B. (1996). Calcium sparks and $[Ca^{2+}]_i$ waves in cardiac myocytes. *Am J Physiol*, *270*, C148-C159.

[11] Cui, J. & Kaandorp, J. A. (2006). Mathematical modeling of calcium homeostasis in yeast cells. *Cell Calcium*, *39*, 337-348.

[12] Cui, J., & Kaandorp, J. A. (2008). Simulating complex calcium-calcineurin signaling network. In M. Bubak, G. D. van Albada, J. Dongarra, & P. M. A. Sloot (Eds.), *Lecture Notes in Computer Science* (Vol. 5103, pp. 110-119). Heidelberg: Springer-Verlag Berlin.

[13] Cui, J., Kaandoorp, J., Ositelu, O. O., Beaudry, V., Knight, A., Nanfack, Y. F. & Cunningham, K. W. (2009). Simulating calcium influx and free calcium concentrations in yeast. *Cell Calcium*, *45*, 123-132.

[14] Cui, J., Kaandorp, J., Sloot, P. M. A., Thiagarajan, P. S., Lloyd, C. M. & Filatov, M. (2009). Calcium homeostasis and signaling in yeast cells and cardiac myocytes. *FEMS Yeast Reasearch*, in press.

[15] Dolinski, K. & Botstein, D. (2007). Orthology and functional conservation in eukaryotes. *Annu Rev Genet*, *41*, 465-507.

[16] Dolmetsch, R. E., Lewis, R. S., Goodnow, C. C. & Healy, J. I. (1997) Differential activation of transcription factors induced by Ca^{2+} response amplitude and duration. *Nature*, *386*, 855 - 858.

[17] Finkelstein, A., Hetherington, J., Li, L., Margoninski, O., Saffrey, P., Seymour, R. & Warner, A. (2004). Computational challenges of systems biology. *Computer*, *37*, 26-33.

[18] **Frey, N., McKinsey, T. A. & Olson** E. N. (2000). Decoding calcium signals involved in cardiac growth and function. ***Nat Med***, ***6***, **1221 - 1227.**

[19] Groff, J. R. & Smith, G. D. (2008). Ryanodine receptor allosteric coupling and the dynamics of calcium sparks. *Biophys J*, *95*, 135-154.

[20] Hallhuber, M., Burkard, N., Wu, R., Buch, M. H., Engelhardt, S., Hein, L., Neyses, L., Schuh, K. & Ritter, O. (2006). Inhibition of nuclear import of calcineurin prevents myocardial hypertrophy. *Circ Res*, *99*, 626 - 635.

[21] Hayashi, M. & Lee, J. D. (2004). Role of the BMK1/ERK5 signaling pathway: lessons from knockout mice. *J Mol Med*, *82*, 800-808.

[22] Heineke, J. & Molkentin, J. D. (2006). Regulation of cardiac hypertrophy by intracellular signaling pathways. *Nat Rev Mol Cell Biol*, *7*, 589-600.

[23] Hilioti, Z., Gallagher, D. A., Low-Nam, S. T., Ramaswamy, P., Gajer, P., Kingsbury, T. J., Birchwood, C. J., Levchenko, A. & Cunningham,

K. W. (2004). GSK-3 kinases enhance calcineurin signaling by phosphorylation of RCNs. *Genes & Dev*, *18*, 35 - 47.

[24] Kingsbury, T. K. & Cunningham, K. W. (2000). A conserved family of calcineurin regulators. *Genes & Dev*, *14*, 1595-1604.

[25] Kishi, T., Ikeda, A., Nagao, R. & Koyama, N. (2007). The SCF[Cdc4] ubiquitin ligase regulates calcineurin signaling through degradation of phosphorylated Rcn1, an inhibitor of calcineurin. *Proc Natl Acad Sci U S A*, *104*, 17418-23.

[26] Koninck, P. D. & Schulman, H. (1998). Sensitivity of CaM kinase II to the frequency of Ca^{2+} oscillations. *Science*, *279*, 227 - 230.

[27] Liao, W., Wang, S., Han, C. & Zhang, Y. (2005). 14-3-3 Proteins regulate glycogen synthase3β phosphorylation and inhibit cardiomyocyte hypertrophy. *FEBS J*, *272*, 1845-1854.

[28] Lloyd, C. M., Lawson, J. R., Hunter, P. J. & Nielsen, P. F. (2008) The CellML model repository. *Bioinformatics*, *24*, 2122-2123.

[29] Mackenzie, L., Roderick, H. L., Berridge, M. J., Conway, S. J. & Bootman, M. D. (2004). The spatial pattern of atrial cardiomyocyte calcium signalling modulates contraction. *J Cell Sci*, *117*, 6327-6337.

[30] Marks, A. R. (2003). Calcium and the heart: a question of life and death. *J Clin Invest*, *111*, 597-600.

[31] Niederer, S. A., Hunter, P. J. & Smith, N. P. (2006). A quantitative analysis of cardiac myocyte relaxation: a simulation study. *Biophys J*, *90*, 1697-1722.

[32] Petersen, O.H., Michalak, M. & Verkhratsky, A. (2005). Calcium signalling: past, present and future. *Cell Calcium*, *38*, 161-169.

[33] Putney, JW Jr (Ed). Calcium signaling. 2nd Edition. Boca Raton: CRC Press; 2005.

[34] Rudolf, R., Mongillo, M., Rizzuto, R. & Pozzan, T. (2003). Looking forward to seeing calcium. *Nat Rev Mol Cell Biol*, *4*, 579-586.

[35] Scrase-Field, S. A. M. G. & Knight, M. R. (2003) Calcium: just a chemical switch? *Curr Opin Plant Biol*, *6*, 500-506.

[36] Shannon, T. R., Wang, F., Puglisi, J., Webber, C. & Bers, D. M. (2004). A mathematical treatment of integrated Ca dynamics within the ventricular myocyte. *Biophys J*, *87*, 3351-3371.

[37] Shin, S.-Y., Choo, S.-M., Kim, D., Baek, S. J., Wolkenhauer, O. & Cho, K.-H. (2006). Switching feedback mechanisms realize the dual role of RCAN in the regulation of calcineurin activity. *FEBS Lett*, *580*, 5965-5973.

[38] Sipido, K. R. & Eisner, D. (2005). Something old, something new: changing views on the cellular mechanisms of heart failure. *Cardio Res*, *68*, 167-174.

[39] Sobie, E. A., Dilly, K. W., dos Santos Cruz, J., Lederer, W. J. & Jafri, M. S. (2002). Termination of cardiac Ca^{2+} sparks: an investigative mathematical model of calcium-induced calcium release. *Biophys J*, *83*, 59-78.

[40] Takeishi, Y., Huang, Q., Abe, J.-I., Glassman, M., Che, W., Lee, J.-D., Kawakatsu, H., Lawrence, E. G., Hoit, B. D., Berk, B. C. & Walsh, R. A. (2001). Src and multiple MAP kinase activation in cardiac hypertrophy and congestive heart failure under chronic pressure-overload: Comparison with acute mechanical stretch. *J Mol Cell Cardio*, *33*, 1637-1648.

[41] Thomine, S. (2001). Cracking the calcium code. *Trends Plant Sci*, *6*, 501.

[42] Vega, R. B., Bassel-Duby, R. & Olson, E. N. (2003). Control of Cardiac growth and function by calcineurin signaling. *J Biol Chem*, *278*, 36981-36984.

[43] Vega, R. B., Rothermel, B. A., Weinheimer, C. J., Kovacs, A., Naseem, R. H., Bassel-Duby, R., Williams, R. S. & Olson, E. N. (2003). Dual roles of modulatory calcineurin-interacting protein 1 in cardiac hypertrophy. *Proc Natl Acad Sci USA*, *100*, 669-674.

[44] Weber, C. R., Piacentino, V., Ginsburg, K. S., Houser, S. R. & Bers, D. M. (2002). Na^+-Ca^{2+} exchange current and submembrane $[Ca^{2+}]$ during the cardiac action potential. *Circ Res*, *90*, 182-189.

APPENDIX

The detailed equations of the model are as follows:

$$\frac{dCaM(t)}{dt} = -k_1 Ca^4 CaM(t) + k_2 CaMCa(t)$$

$$\frac{dCaMCa(t)}{dt} = k_1 Ca^4 CaM(t) - k_2 CaMCa(t) - k_3 CaMCa(t)CaNa(t) + k_4 CaNc^*(t)$$

$$\frac{dCaNa(t)}{dt} = -k_3 CaMCa(t)CaNa(t) + k_4 CaNc^*(t)$$

$$\frac{dComp1(t)}{dt} = -k_6 Comp1(t) + k_5 RCAN(t)CaNc^*(t)$$

$$\frac{dComp2(t)}{dt} = -k_{20} Comp2(t) + k_{19} RCANpp(t)P1433(t)$$

$$\frac{dComp3(t)}{dt} = -k_{28} Comp3(t) + k_{27} NFATpa(t)P1433(t)$$

$$\frac{dMRNA(t)}{dt} = k_{41} NFATn(t) - k_{42} MRNA(t)$$

$$\frac{dBMK1(t)}{dt} = -k_7 BMK1(t)RCAN(t) + (k_8 + k_9)RCAN \cup BMK1(t)$$

$$\frac{dGSK3\beta c(t)}{dt} = -k_{31} GSK3\beta c(t) + k_{32} GSK3\beta n(t) - k_{13} GSK3\beta c(t)RCANp(t)$$
$$+ (k_{14} + k_{15})RCANp \cup GSK3\beta c(t) - k_{24} GSK3\beta c(t)NFATc(t)$$
$$+ (k_{25} + k_{26})NFATc \cup GSK3\beta c(t)$$

$$\frac{dGSK3\beta n(t)}{dt} = k_{31} GSK3\beta c(t) - k_{32} GSK3\beta n(t) - k_{38} GSK3\beta n(t)NFATn(t)$$
$$+ (k_{39} + k_{40})NFATn \cup GSK3\beta n(t)$$

$$\frac{dRCAN(t)}{dt} = k_{43} MRNA(t) - (\ln 2/15)RCAN(t) + k_6 Comp1(t) - k_7 BMK1(t)RCAN(t)$$
$$+ k_8 RCAN \cup BMK1(t) + k_{12} RCANp \cup CaNc^*(t) - k_5 RCAN(t)CaNc^*(t)$$

$$\frac{dRCANp(t)}{dt} = -k_{13} GSK3\beta c(t)RCANp(t) + k_{14} RCANp \cup GSK3\beta c(t) + k_9 RCAN \cup BMK1(t)$$
$$+ k_{18} RCANpp \cup CaNc^*(t) + k_{11} RCANp \cup CaNc^*(t) - k_{10} RCANp(t)CaNc^*(t)$$

$$\frac{dRCANpp(t)}{dt} = k_{20} Comp2(t) + k_{15} RCANp \cup GSK3\beta c(t) - k_{19} RCANpp(t)P1433(t)$$
$$+ k_{17} RCANpp \cup CaNc^*(t) - k_{16} RCANpp(t)CaNc^*(t)$$

$$\frac{dRCANp \cup GSK3\beta c(t)}{dt} = k_{13} GSK3\beta c(t)RCANp(t) - (k_{14} + k_{15})RCANp \cup GSK3\beta c(t)$$

$$\frac{dRCAN \cup BMK1(t)}{dt} = k_7 BMK1(t)RCAN(t) - (k_8 + k_9)RCAN \cup BMK1(t)$$

$$\frac{dNFATc(t)}{dt} = -k_{29} NFATc(t) - k_{24} GSK3\beta c(t)NFATc(t) + k_{25} NFATc \cup GSK3\beta c(t)$$
$$+ k_{23} NFATpc \cup CaNc^*(t)$$

$$\frac{dNFATc \cup GSK3\beta c(t)}{dt} = k_{24} GSK3\beta c(t)NFATc(t) - (k_{25} + k_{26})NFATc \cup GSK3\beta c(t)$$

$$\frac{dNFATn(t)}{dt} = k_{29}NFATc(t) - k_{38}GSK3\beta n(t)NFATn(t) + k_{39}NFATn \cup GSK3\beta n(t)$$

$$+ k_{37}NFATpn \cup CaNn^*(t)$$

$$\frac{dNFATn \cup GSK3\beta n(t)}{dt} = k_{38}GSK3\beta n(t)NFATn(t) - (k_{39} + k_{40})NFATn \cup GSK3\beta n(t)$$

$$\frac{dNFATpc(t)}{dt} = k_{28}Comp3(t) + k_{26}NFATc \cup GSK3\beta c(t) + k_{30}NFATpn(t)$$

$$- k_{27}NFATpc(t) \cup P1433(t) + k_{22}NFATpc \cup CaNc^*(t) - k_{21}NFATpc(t)CaNc^*(t)$$

$$\frac{dNFATpn(t)}{dt} = k_{40}NFATn \cup GSK3\beta n(t) - k_{30}NFATpn(t)$$

$$+ k_{36}NFATpn \cup CaNn^*(t) - k_{35}NFATpn(t)CaNn^*(t)$$

$$\frac{dP1433(t)}{dt} = k_{20}Comp2(t) + k_{28}Comp3(t) - k_{19}RCANpp(t)P1433(t) - k_{27}NFATpc(t)P1433(t)$$

$$\frac{dRCANpp \cup CaNc^*(t)}{dt} = -(k_{17} + k_{18})RCANpp \cup CaNc^*(t) + k_{16}RCANpp(t)CaNc^*(t)$$

$$\frac{dRCANp \cup CaNc^*(t)}{dt} = -(k_{11} + k_{12})RCANp \cup CaNc^*(t) + k_{10}RCANp(t)CaNc^*(t)$$

$$\frac{dNFATpc \cup CaNc^*(t)}{dt} = -(k_{22} + k_{23})NFATpc \cup CaNc^*(t) + k_{21}NFATpc(t)CaNc^*(t)$$

$$\frac{dNFATpn \cup CaNn^*(t)}{dt} = -(k_{36} + k_{37})NFATpn \cup CaNn^*(t) + k_{35}NFATpn(t)CaNn^*(t)$$

$$\frac{dCaNc^*(t)}{dt} = k_3CaMCa(t)CaNc(t) + k_6Comp1(t) + (k_{11} + k_{12})RCANp \cup CaNc^*(t)$$

$$- k_{10}RCANp(t)CaNc^*(t) + (k_{17} + k_{18})RCANpp \cup CaNc^*(t) - k_{16}RCANpp(t)CaNc^*(t)$$

$$+ (k_{22} + k_{23})NFATpc \cup CaNc^*(t) - k_{21}NFATpc(t)CaNc^*(t) - k_{33}CaNc^*(t) - k_4CaNc^*(t)$$

$$- k_5RCAN(t)CaNc^*(t) + k_{34}CaNn^*(t)$$

$$\frac{dCaNn^*(t)}{dt} = (k_{36} + k_{37})NFATpn \cup CaNn^*(t) - k_{35}NFATpn(t)CaNn^*(t) + k_{33}CaNc^*(t)$$

$$- k_{34}CaNn^*(t)$$

Where parameter Ca denotes the cytosolic calcium concentration (please note that here $RCAN \cup BMK1(0)$ denotes the initial concentration of intermediate complex formed by RCAN and BMK1. For the meaning of the relevant variables, please see the abbreviations and synonyms listed in the legend of Figure 2).

The initial condition used for the simulations is as follows (Units are in μM):

$BMK1(0) = 0.012, MRNA(0) = 3.33*10^{-4}, CaM(0) = 25.2, CaMCa(0) = 7.88*10^{-7},$

$CaNc(0) = 0.91, CaNc^*(0) = 0.0275, CaNn^*(0) = 0.0568, Comp1(0) = 5.21*10^{-3},$

$Comp2(0) = 0.283, Comp3(0) = 0.014, GSK3\beta c(0) = 0.17, GSK3\beta n(0) = 0.339,$

$RCAN(0) = 2.15*10^{-4}, RCANp(0) = 7.76*10^{-3}, RCANpp(0) = 0.0798, P1433(0) = 0.708,$

$NFATc(0) = 2*10^{-5}, NFATn(0) = 4.99*10^{-4}, NFATpc(0) = 4.94*10^{-3}, NFATpn(0) = 8.01*10^{-5},$

$NFATc \cup GSK3\beta c(0) = 1.36*10^{-6}, NFATn \cup GSK3\beta n(0) = 8.46*10^{-5},$

$RCANp \cup GSK3\beta c(0) = 1.1*10^{-3}, RCAN \cup BMK1(0) = 2.14*10^{-5},$

$RCANpp \cup CaNc^*(0) = 1.1*10^{-3}, RCANp \cup CaNc^*(0) = 1.07*10^{-4},$

$NFATpn \cup CaNn^*(0) = 2.27*10^{-6}, NFATpc \cup CaNc^*(0) = 8.15*10^{-5}$

(Please note that this initial condition is a selected steady state for simulating the normally growing heart cells with parameter $Ca = 0.05\mu M$).

The simulation of the stimuli is as follows:

1. PO stimulus is simulated by simultaneously setting $Ca = 0.2\mu M$ and increasing $BMK1(0)$ from 0.012µM to 1.2µM.

2. The stimulus of CaN* overexpression is simulated by simultaneously setting $Ca = 0.4\mu M$ and increasing $CaNc^*(0)$ from 0.0275µM to 0.825µM.

In: Congestive Heart Failure...   ISBN: 978-1-60876-677-2
Editors: J. E. García et al. pp. 129-151   © 2010 Nova Science Publishers, Inc.

Chapter 6

RIGHT VENTRICULAR FAILURE IN CARDIAC SURGERY

Tadashi Omoto and Takeo Tedoriya

Department of Surgery, Division of Thoracic and Cardiovascular Surgery
Showa University Tokyo, Japan

I. INTRODUCTION

Right ventricular (RV) function plays an important role in the clinical outcome of cardiac surgery. RV failure observed in the operating room is notable for the bulging and distention of the RV free wall [1]. When it occurs in the intra-operative period, RV failure is associated with failure to wean from cardiopulmonary bypass and the need for massive inotropic and mechanical support. Insufficient protection for RV remains to be an important limitation in current cardioplegic technique, either antegrade or retrograde [2], particularly in the context of RV hypertrophy and coronary artery disease [3]. The RV has shown to be a risk factor of postoperative early mortality of valve surgery, coronary surgery, cardiac transplantation and implantation of left ventricular assist device (LVAD).

RV dysfunction after mitral valve operation is associated with high pulmonary vascular resistance, secondary tricuspid valve insufficiency and a decrease in interventricular interaction resulted from LV dysfunction [4]. Pinzani *et al* demonstrated a significance of RV dysfunction for the prognosis of mitral or mitrla-aortic valve disease [5]. They studied 221 patients without RV failure and 161 patients with RV failure and demonstrated that patients with RV failure had more than double higher early and late mortality. The hemodynamic alterations that occur as a result of heart transplantation or LVAD implantation have placed new emphasis on RV function in cardiac surgery. RV failure after heart transplantation is associated with high pulmonary vascular resistance in the recipient as a result of long-standing congestive heart failure, size mismatch between donor and recipient, and primary graft failure [6]. Chang *et al* reported significances of mild, moderate and severe pulmonary hypertension for heart transplantation, and demonstrated that severe pulmonary hypertension was associated with higher mortality within the first year [7]. They also demonstrated that each 1 wood unit increase in preoperative pulmonary vascular resistance showed a trend toward increased mortality in heart transplantation recipients with mild to moderate preoperative pulmonary hypertension. RV dysfunction after LVAD implantation is associated with changes in interventricular interaction [8,9]. Loss of LV performance may deteriorate RV performance in those patients whose RV performance had been dependent on interventricular interaction. Left-ward shift of the septal wall results in an increase in RV end-diastolic volume. After LVAD implantation, pulmonary vascular resistance decreases, so that RV systolic pressure decreases at the same stroke volume. In pressure-volume curve, end-diastolic volume is right-ward shifted after LVAD implantation (Figure 1).

2. DIFFERENCES BETWEEN THE RV AND LV

RV failure cannot be understood simply by extrapolating data and experiences from LV failure. LV must generate a high pressure to overcome higher vascular resistance and allow appropriate distribution of systemic perfusion with differences in peripheral resistance. The RV ejects into a more uniform and compliant pulmonary vascular bed, generating lower pressure. Between the RV and LV, there are many different intrinsic factors. And these differences may have implications in the assessment and treatment of patients with RV failure. The RV and the LV originate from different progenitor cells and different sites. The primary heart field gives rise to the atrial chambers and the LV, whereas the cells of the anterior heart field develop into the outflow tract and the RV [10].

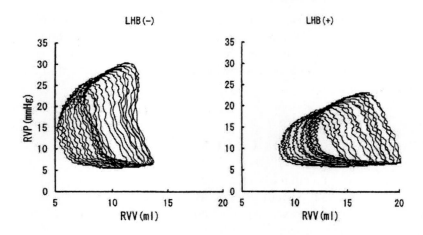

Figure 1. Right ventricular pressure-volume loops obtained by changing preload. LHB(-), Without left heart bypass; LHB(+), with left heart bypass; RVP, right ventricular pressure; RV, right ventricular volume by conductance catheter. (Kitano M et al. J Thorac Cardiovasc Surg 1995;109:796-803).

Two ventricles are different in fiber orientation within the ventricular walls, chamber geometry, myosin isoenzyme distribution which affects the speed of contractile shortening. Creatine kinase activity is lower in the RV [11], and ratio of mitochondria to myofibrils is lower in the RV[12]. Coronary blood flow is lower in RV tissue and oxygen consumption per tissue is also lower in RV tissue [13]. Composition of myosin isozyme V1 is higher in RV than LV, which results in quicker contractile shortening in the RV [14]. The RV muscle has a more rapid speed of shortening at light loads which correlates with differences in isomyosin distribution with LV muscle. The complex collagen and elastic network of the RV micro-architecture may play an important role in the wall stress-sarcomere length relationship [15,16].

The difference in configuration between the two ventricles is demonstrated by a transverse section. The LV chamber is an ellipsoidal sphere surrounded by relatively thick musculature, and the RV has a crescent-shaped chamber and a thin wall. The RV has a large sinus portion that surrounds and supports the tricuspid valve and outlet portion which supports the pulmonary valve. The septal surface of the RV is divided into an inlet portion, a trabecular portion and an outlet portion. The inlet and trabecular portion, consisting of the tricuspid valve and the travecular muscles of the anterior and inferior walls, directs entering blood anteriorly, inferiorly and to the left at an angle of 60 degree to the outflow tract [17]. The outflow tract has a thick muscle, *the crista supuraventricularis,* which ejects blood into the pulmonary artery. The LV wall is arranged in three different layers: subepicardial, middle and subendocardial. These distinctions are made by a change in direction of the muscle fibers. The middle layer, showing a circumferential pattern in the LV, is not present in the RV.

3. RV FUNCTION

Studies of RV function have been developed as application of indices of LV function. In 1954, Sarnoff *et al* demonstrated in dogs that in any given physiologic state there was a consistent and reproducible correlation between atrial pressure and ventricular stroke volume on both the RV and LV (Frank-Starling's principle) [18]. Previous investigations had viewed the RV as a passive conduit for systemic venous return rather than an active pump [19,20]. This concept was derived from experimental findings that the RV free wall could be extensively damaged without decreasing cardiac output or significantly distorting RV systolic pressure. Routinely measured indices of function such as ejection fraction or dP/dt are all load dependent. Pressure-volume analysis allows derivation of load-independent indices of LV function, such as the end-systolic pressure volume relationship or the preload recruitable stroke work relationship. End-systolic pressure-volume relationship was first described by Suga and Sagawa for the LV [21]. In these studies, they determined that the slope of the end-systolic pressure-volume relationship was insensitive to changes in preload and afterload but sensitive to changes in contractile state of the LV.

Volume of LV has been measured in experimental or clinical settings by cineangiography, radioisotope imaging or echocardiography. Many experiments for investigation of RV function have been hampered by the difficulty of measuring the instantaneous volume of the RV due to its complex geometry. The LV cavity is ellipsoid in shape and RV cavity is roughly triangular in shape. The local distending pressure-stress relationship is hererogeneous along the RV walls and can change as a result of septal shift. Conductance measurements of absolute RV volume provided an instantaneous volume index better validated for the LV [22].

Maughan *et al* demonstrated pressure-volume relationship in the RV performance, measuring RV volume by the use of a water-filled, thin latex balloon [23]. The isovolumic contraction period in the RV is short, and blood is ejected as pressure is declining at end-systole. In their study, RV contractile performance based on interpretation of the pressure-volume loop demonstrated that there is a strong relationship between global RV stroke work (pressure-volume loop area) and end-diastolic volume; the lineality of preload recruitable stroke work relationship [23]. Development of the ellipsoidal shell subtraction model had enabled actual RV volume analysis and assessment of unidimensional indexes in the RV [24]. RV free wall contractility has been studied in pressure-length analysis. Morris *et al* demonstrated that the regional stroke work vs. end-diastolic length relation is a reliable index of regional ventricular function in the right and left ventricle [25].

Figure 2 shows representative pressure-length loops of the RV. RV free wall regional stroke work was calculated as RV pressure-dimension loop area. The shape of pressure-length loops is triangular in the RV and quadrangular in the LV. This characteristic is the reflection of end-systolic performance of the RV. In isolated canine hearts, the relationship between RV free wall segment length and RV volume is linear.

Despite those improvements in quantifying RV contractility, the assessment in RV function has been limited because of the following problems.

1. Interventricular interaction; Unidemensional indexes which are calculated by RV pressure-volume (length) loop is the interactive effect of LV volume on RV shape.
2. The RV is more susceptible to afterload, i.e. high pulmonary artery pressure. When RV preload or stroke volume was held constant, RV free wall segment length increased or decreased with changes in RV afterload. Because the RV is thin walled, transmural wall stress also increases dramatically.
3. Change in preload (elevated filling pressure) alters coronary perfusion which may complicate the assessment of RV contractility [26]. Volume loading to examine the RV pressure-volume loop may be limited by impairment of RV myocardial blood flow.

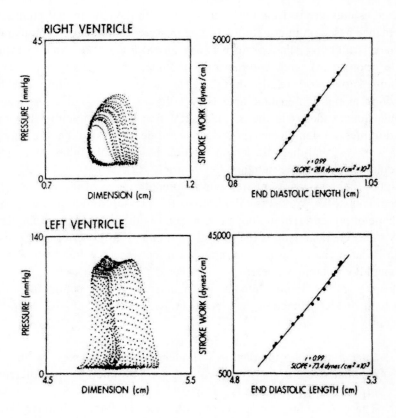

Figure 2. Representative pressure-length loops of the left and right ventricle. The linear relationships were shown between regional stroke work vs. end-diastolic length in both ventricles. (Morris JJ et al, J Thorac Cardiovasc Surg 1986;91:879-887).

[Negative Intrathoracic Pressure in Early Diastole in the RV]

A negative pressure is often measured in the human RV during early diastole, reflecting a negative intrathoracic pressure [27]. Sabbah *et al* demonstrated in dogs with the chest open, a negative RV pressure during early diastole [28]. When the chest is open, RV pressure during early diastole was less negative than when the chest was closed. This difference may relate to a change of right atrial pressure. The mechanism of ventricular suction is speculative.

Isolated RV model

The RV pressure-volume curve is influenced by LV performance. RV myocardial perfusion is associated with LV afterload. Thus, in order to evaluate RV pressure-volume relationship during changing RV preload and afterload, left ventricular performance and coronary perfusion should be held constant.

Omoto *et al* developed an isolate RV model to show different RV performance between volume overload and pressure overload [29]. In experimental canine model, coronary perfusion pressure was held constant using cardiopulmonary bypass with left ventricle unloaded, causing interventricular interaction as zero and RV preload and afterload were regulated (Figure 3A).

(A)

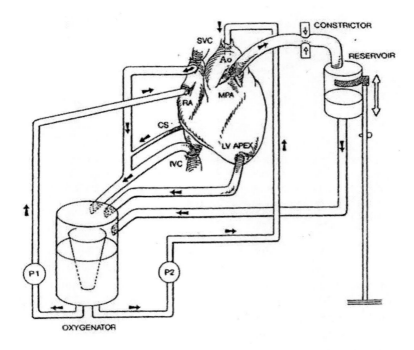

Figure 3 (Continued).

(B)

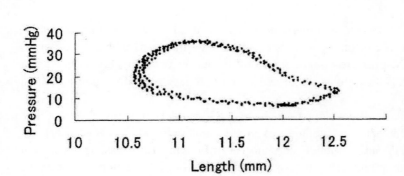

(C)

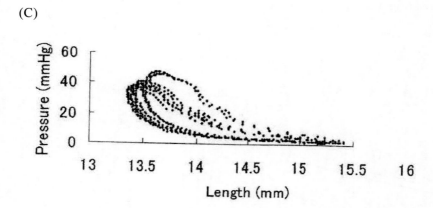

Figure 3. (A) Isolated right ventricular model. Ao: aorta, SVC: superior vena cava, RA: right atrium, IVC: inferior vena cava, MPA: main pulmonary artery, LV: left ventricle, P1: pump 1, P2: pump 2(Omoto T, Thorac Cardiovasc Surg 2002;50:16-20). (B) Pressure-length loops (changes in stroke volume). (C) Pressure-length loops (changes in afterload).

From superior vena cava, inferior vena cava and coronary sinus, venous drainage was performed. Via left ventricular apex, left ventricle was completely drained. Main pulmonary artery was drained into reservoir and RV pressure was regulated by constrictor and height of the reservoir. RV preload was regulated by pump1. Aortic pressure and coronary artery pressure were controlled at 60 mmHg by another perfusion pump. Using this experimental model, (a) functional analysis could be performed without ventricular interaction from the left ventricle, (b) RV preload and afterload could be regulated, and (c) coronary perfusion could be regulated.

First, RV systolic pressure held constant. RV preload was increased by several stages. However RV stroke work and end-diastolic length were not linearly increase (Figure 3B). In cases with pressure overload, contrasting results were showed. Increase in afterload increases RV stroke work under constant preload (Figure 3C). The data showed that there were linear relationships between RV stroke work vs. RV end-diastolic length as well as RV stroke work vs. RV peak pressure. These results lead to the concept that the ventricular function curve, which has ventricular stroke work as y-axis and preload as x-axis, could be better replaced by afterload as x-axis when we evaluate RV function.

RV function curve could be variable depending on pulmonary vascular compliance and myocardial changes. Compensated chronic volume overloaded RV may show that optimal contractility of the RV is rather higher RV systolic pressure. RV dysfunction after ischemic reperfusion injury showed a decrease in RV stroke work at rather lower RV systolic pressure.

This experimental model avoided this confounding issue by using an unloaded left ventricle, thus minimizing the contributor of the interventricular septum to RV function. This permitted our experimental model to focus only on RV free wall function and not global RV performance. Although not examined in this study, preservation of left ventricle and interventricular septal function may contribute improvements in RV global function after ischemia in relevant clinical settings.

Interventricular interaction

Previous studies have shown that loading on one ventricle may alter compliance, configuration or performance of the other ventricle [30,31]. This so-called ventricular interdependence is defined by the forces that are transmitted from one ventricle to the other ventricle through the myocardium and pericardium, independent of neural, humoral or circulatory effects [32]. Abnormalities of RV function are not only attributed to primary abnormalities of RV myocardium but also to LV dysfunction.

Interventricular interaction has been classified into two categories: diastolic and systolic ventricular interaction. The diastolic pressure-volume relationship of one ventricle is dependent on the degree of the other (diastolic ventricular interaction). Contraction of one ventricle influences the performance of the other ventricle (systolic ventricular interation). It has been thought that the influence of left ventricular performance on RV performance is much more than the influence of RV performance on left ventricular performance.

Diastolic Ventricular Interaction

The volume or pressure in one ventricle can directly influence the volume and pressure in the other ventricle. Yamaguchi *et al* observed that increasing left ventricular volume displaced the interventricular septum toward the RV and alters the RV pressure-volume relationship in canine hearts [33].

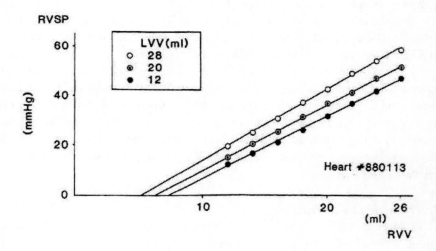

Figure 4. Graph showing the example of right ventricular end-systolic pressure-volume relation under three left ventricular volume (LVV) levels (12, 20, and 20ml). Right ventricular end-systolic pressure-volume relation was determined using right ventricular peak systolic pressure (RVSP) of isovolumic contraction. When LVV was increased from 12 to 28 ml, the slope of the end-systolic pressure-volume relation was augmented and the volume intercept was decreased. RVV. Right ventricular volume. (Yamaguchi S et al. Circulation Research 1989;65:623-631ʳ)

Figure 4 shows the relationship between RV systolic pressure and RV volume, at different left ventricular volume (12, 20 and 28ml). With an increase in left ventricular volume, RV end-systolic pressure volume relation shifted upward and leftward shift. They concluded that it was explained by the alteration of end-diastolic length in RV free wall that occurred with constant RV volume, probably due to the deformation of RV becoming more crescent in shape. End-diastolic pressure-volume relationship of the RV depends on that of the LV. Increased distention of LV during diastole alters the compliance and geometry of the RV.

Systolic Ventricular Interaction

Experimental studies have shown that systolic ventricular interaction is an immediate effect. Woodart *et al* showed rapid that withdrawal or injections into the LV caused immediate changes in RV pressure and volume [34]. Feneley *et al* demonstrated that acute increments in LV afterload decrease the work output from the RV at any given end-diastolic volume (preload), a direct, negative systolic ventricular interaction [35]. Right-ward systolic displacement of the interventricular septum due to the increase in LV systolic pressure during increased LV afterload contributes to this interaction [36]. The increased radius of RV free wall curvature would result in greater systolic stress for the same developed pressure with a consequent reduction in systolic shortening.

Damiano *et al* examined electrically isolated RV free wall preparation allowed for wide variations in the timing interval between RV and LV contractions [37]. Double-peaked waveforms for RV pressure and pulmonary arterial blood flow occurred over a wide range of pacing intervals between the RV and LV. These two waveforms were related to RV and LV contractions. For LV pressure, the LV component was significantly larger than the RV component. RV systolic pressure and pulmonary artery blood flow were composed of both RV and LV components, with the LV component dominating.

The RV begins to eject almost without isovolumic systolic contraction. The pressure in the LV is increasing rapidly, which increase RV pressure to start RV ejection through interventricular interaction. Yamaguchi *et al* obsereved that the duration of RV ejection was decreased by a sudden decrease in LV afterload [38]. This phenomenon was directly related to the length of LV systole. The RV begins to eject almost without an isovolumetric systolic contraction and continues to eject after end-systole.

The septum is the key element in interventricular interaction. Alteration in septal position changes with alteration in systolic loading condition. For instance, pulmonary artery constriction causes a leftward septal shift. The position of the interventricular septum depends on (1) the transseptal pressure gradient, (2) geometry and fiber orientation of the septum, and (c) contractility of the RV and the LV. The septum and its position are not the sole mechanism for ventricular interdependence. Ventricular interdependence causes overall ventricular deformation and is probably best explained by the balance of forces at the interventricular sulcus, the material proterties and cardiac dimensions [39].

Effects of LVAD Implantation on RV Function

Studies of LVAD implantation had demonstrated important effects of interventricular interaction on RV function [40]. After LVAD implantation, decreasing LV preload will decrease pulmonary artery pressure. RV filling is increased by the increased cardiac output with LVAD. RV filling is further increased by leftward shift of the interventricular septum. Figure 1 shows RV performance during left heart bypass [40]. RV end-diastolic volume was increased and RV systolic pressure decreases after left heart bypass. If the RV keeps stroke volume constant, larger preload or volume expansion is required for larger end-diastolic volume. Pathological RV with severe RV hypertrophy, RV dilatation or secondary tricuspid regurgitation is unable to respond to this hemodynamic requirement. Furthermore, after LVAD support, the reduced LV systolic assistance leads to a decrease in RV systolic function. Reduced RV contractility due to global ischemia during LVAD implantation may deteriorate this loss of systolic ventricular interaction.

RV Afterload

Compared with the left ventricle, RV is susceptible to acute pressure overload. Increase in RV afterload results in vasodilation of coronary arteries, however further increase in RV afterload results in vasoconstriction of coronary arteries and RV ischemia occurs. Increase in myocardial perfusion pressure reverses RV ischemia. Vlahakes *et al* studied RV performance and

RV myocardial coronary perfusion during increase in RV afterload in canines [41].

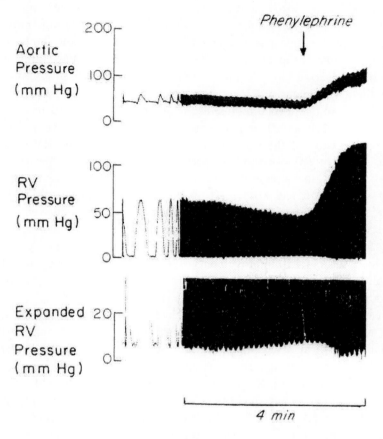

Figure 5. Hemodynamic example of the effects of phenylephrine in acute right ventricular (RV) failure in a preparation with a closed pericardium All three recordings were taken at a slow paper speed (Reprinted by permission of the publisher from Vlahakes GJ et al. Circulation 1981;63:87-95).

Figure 5 shows systemic arteral blood pressure and RV pressure during pulmonary artery constriction. PA is gradually constricted until aortic pressure declines and RV pressure falls (RV failure). During increased RV systolic pressure, the determinants of RV oxygen requirements increase. At the onset of RV failure, there was no coronary vasodilation reserve indicating RV myocardial ischemia. Infusion of phenylephrine raised systemic blood pressure, and hence myocardial perfusion pressure; RV failure reversed as shown by increased cardiac output and RV systolic pressure (recovered RV failure).

Vlahakes *et al* also showed tissue creatine phosphate and ATP concentration during acute pressure overloading [41]. During pressure overloading creatine phosphate and ATP were held constant, however a decrease in creatine phosphate and ATP occurs during RV failure. Infusion of phenylephrine reversed biological deterioration. During increased RV systolic pressure, the determinants of RV oxygen requirements increase. In contrast to the LV, a pressure overload stimulus results in a marked, selective increase in resting transmural blood flow per gram of the RV [42]. Since increased systolic compression of the intramural coronary vessels during RV systolic hypertension effectively decreases the perfusion pressure gradient between the aorta and the RV, an increase in diastolic myocardial blood flow occurs by coronary vasodilation and a decrease in coronary vascular resistance [43]. Previous studies concerning coronary perfusion and the right ventricular afterload showed that a decrease in coronary blood flow during acute RV pressure loading is due to vasoconstriction which is mediated by alpha-adrenergic effects [44,45]. Improvements of RV ischemia are demonstrated by phenylephrine which increases coronary perfusion pressure or adenosine which decreases coronary vascular resistance (Figure 5).

Increase in RV stroke work was associated with a rise in end-diastolic pressure and volume, which indicates the utilization of the Frank-Starling mechanism as a form of adaptation to increased afterload. Fourie PR *et al* investigated the ventricular/vascular coupling of the RV under normal and afterloading condition [46]. RV contractility was obtained by calculating the end-systolic elastance (Ees) and the effective pulmonary arterial elastance (Ea). The Ees-Ea relation yields a direct assessment of ventricular-arterial coupling efficiency. With an increase in afterload, RV stroke work increases (Ees>Ea). A further increase in afterload will result in a decrease in stroke work (Ees<Ea), i.e. RV failure (Figure 6). The maximum RV stroke work corresponded to a mean pulmonary artery pressure of 30-40 mmHg in their experiments. In clinical practice the catecholamine to increase RV contractility restores the match between the RV and afterload where Ees-Ea coupling is maintained. The adaptation of the RV to its afterload conditions not only depends on the Frank-Starling mechanism but seems also to be regulated by some inherent ability of this ventricle to match the physical factors responsible for pulmonary vascular input impedance [47,48].

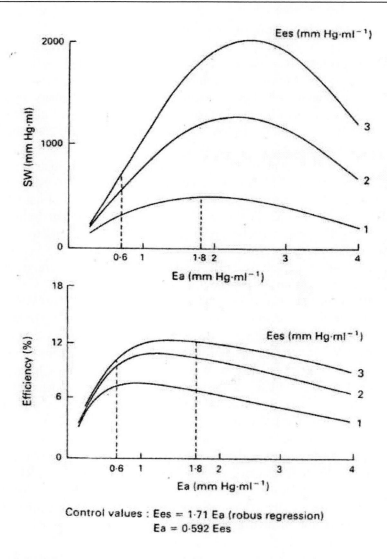

Control values : Ees = 1·71 Ea (robus regression)
Ea = 0·592 Ees

Figure 6. Relation between vascular bed resistance (R) and stroke work (SW) for various conditions of arterial compliance (C). Note that the maximum of the SW curve shifts downwards and to the left with a decrease of compliance from 5 to 0.1 ml · mmHg $^{-1}$. The theoretical SW curve obtained by applying the data for the change in compliance obtained from this study lies between the two extremes (C=5 ml · mmHg $^{-1}$ and 0.1 ml · mmHg $^{-1}$) (Fourier PR et al. Cardiovasc Res 1992;26:839-844).

Effects of Global Ischemia on RV Function

Although it is less often studied we will now look at LV, RV performance after global ischemia. Morris *et al* demonstrated RV performance after 20 minutes and 30 minutes of global ischemia using cardiopulmonary bypass [25]. After global ischemia, slope of stroke work vs. end-diastolic length reduced 28% with 20 minutes global ischemia and reduced 32% with 30 minutes global ischemia. X-intercept was right-ward shifted.

Ventricular wall thickness and myocardial edema are attributed to its functional deterioration. The RV is a normally low-pressure system that receives transmural perfusion throughout the cardiac cycle. The normal RV is highly distensible. Changes in distensability of RV after global ischemia, result in changes in end-diastolic pressure and volume relationship. After global ischemia, small changes in RV systolic pressure result in larger increases in end-diastolic volume or depression of RV peak pressure vs. end-diastolic length relationship.

Coronary perfusion alters after global ischemia which changes RV free wall performance under pressure loading. Endothelial dysfunction by ischemic reperfusion injury may worsen myocardial blood flow vs. oxygen requirements. RV coronary vasodilator reserve decreases significantly during high RV pressure overloading states. When RV filling pressure is high, RV pre-capillary arterioles dilate, auto-regulating flow to compensate for increased metabolic demands placed on the myocardium. However, when the vasodilator reserve of the RV coronary bed is unable to compensate for the elevated wall tension and tissue pressures, resulting in decline of coronary flow and RV free wall, ischemia deteriorates. Increased wall tension occurring with RV pressure loading has detrimental effects on blood flow to the RV free wall after global ischemia. Loss of vasodilator reserve results in a mechanical impediment to increasing flow. Under these conditions, RV dysfunction may be related to restriction of myocardial blood flow as well as to myofibrillar over-distention (Figure 7).

As discussed previously, LV component for RV performance is significantly large, so that RV dysfunction after global ischemia is associated with RV myocardial damage and LV myocardial damage as well. Global RV function is the result of variable contributions from the RV free wall, the interventricular interaction, coronary perfusion and pulmonary vascular compliance. Those factors should be evaluated after global ischemia

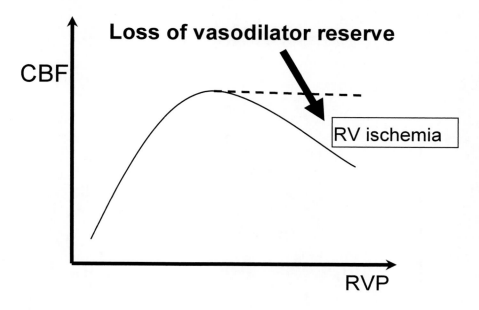

Figure 7. Right ventricular ischemia in high level of right ventricular pressure. CBF; coronary blood flow, RVP right ventricular systolic pressure

Treatment Strategy

RV failure occurred after cardiac operation is often manifested by low cardiac output, low left atrial pressures and high right atrial pressures. Treatment strategy against RV failure after cardiac surgery should be made by first assessing LV function and coronary perfusion, then optimal preload condition and decrease in pulmonary vascular resistance should be considered.

Intravascular volume expansion is a common therapeutic intervention for RV dysfunction and serves to increase the filling pressure. Optimization of RV preload is a major concern in treatment for RV failure. It requires ability to predict the result of rapid fluid infusion. Volume loading or an increase in RV end-diastolic volume, is associated with an increase in RV systolic pressure. RV end-diastolic length is highly associated with RV systolic pressure [29]. Increase in RV preload improves cardiac output when the RV contractility is on the ascending limb of the RV function curve (Figure 8). However volume loading does not improve cardiac output and serves only to distend the RV and raise RV afterload when the RV contractility is on the descending limb of the RV function curve.

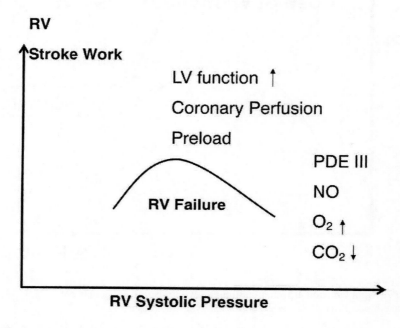

Figure 8. Treatment strategies against RV failure after cardiac operation

Volume loading to treat RV dysfunction may be limited by impairment of RV myocardial blood flow. Vasodilator reserve may be impaired after global ischemia which damages hearts exhibits loss of endothelium dependent factors and reduced nitric oxide even by the current cardiac preservation [49]. Endothelial dysfunction after global ischemia may impair myocardial blood flow at a time when increased oxygen requirements are increased during increased RV afterload. Decrease in myocardial blood flow is caused also by a decrease in LV stroke volume caused by RV dysfunction. Since increased RV systolic and diastolic pressures effectively decrease the perfusion pressure gradient between the aorta and the RV myocardium, RV coronary vasodilator reserve is unable to compensate for the elevated wall tension and tissue pressure, resulting in decline of coronary flow relative to demand and consequent RV free wall ischemia. Improvement of coronary perfusion may reverse RV dysfunction after global ischemia.

If the afterload should be maximal for the RV, additional increment of the afterload (pulmonary vascular resistance) may cause the RV free wall ischemia. Therapy designed to reduce pulmonary vascular resistance (phosphodiesterase III inhibitor, nitric oxide, etc) may be appropriate to increase flow in the setting of increased RV afterload. However, such therapy may also reduce systemic vascular resistance, blood pressure and RV perfusion pressure. Catecholamine may increase coronary perfusion pressure to recover endomyocardial ischemia of the RV, although there have been many arguments that intra-aortic balloon pumping may also increase coronary perfusion.

CONCLUSIONS

Treatment strategy against RV failure after cardiac surgery should be made by the assessment of left ventricular function and coronary perfusion. If the optimal left ventricular function and coronary perfusion are achieved, then optimal preload condition and a decrease in pulmonary vascular resistance should be considered. Volume loading, or increase RV end-diastolic volume, improves cardiac output when RV is on the ascending limb of the Starling curve; however it is associated with an increase in RV afterload which may result in deterioration of RV contractility due to RV ischemia, especially after global ischemia which may cause rightward shift of RV pressure-volume loops.

REFERENCES

[1]   Gonzalez AC, Brandon TA, Fortune RL, et al. Acute right ventricular failure is caused by inadequate right ventricular hypothermia. J Thorac Cardiovasc Surg 1985;89:386

[2]   Ye J, Sun J, Shen J, Gregorash L, Summers R, Salerno TA, Deslauriers R. Does retrograde warm blood cardioplegia provide equal protection to both ventricles?: a magnetic resonance spectroscopy study in pigs. Circulation 1997;96(suppl II): II-210-II-215

[3]   Menasche P, Kucharski K, Mundler O, Veyssie L, Subayi J-B, Le Pimpec F, et al. Adequate preservation of right ventricular function after coronary sinus cardioplegia: a clinical study. Circulation 1989;89:19-24

[4]   Ferrazzi P, McGriffin DC, Kirklin JW, Blackstone EH, Bourge RC.
        Have the results of mitral valve replacement improved? J Thorac
        Cardiovasc Surg 1986;92:186-97

[5]   Pinzani A, de Gevigney G, Pinzani V, Ninet J, Milon H, Delahaye JP.
        Pre- and postoperative right cardiac insufficiency in patients with mitral
        or mitral-aortic valve diseases. Arch Mal Coeur Vaiss 1993;86:27-34

[6]   Szabo G, Sebening C, Hagl C, Tochtermann U, Vahl CF, Hagl S. Right
        ventricular function after brain death: response to an increased afterload.
        Eur J Cardiovasc Surg

[7]   Chang PP, Longenecker JC, Wang NY, Baughman KL, Conte JV, Hare
        JM, Kasper EK. Mild vs. severe pulmonary hypertension before heart
        transplantation: different effects on posttransplantation pulmonary
        hypertension and mortality. J Heart Lung Transplant 2005;24:998-1007

[8]   Park CH, Nishimura K, Kitano M, Matsuda K, Okamoto Y, Ban T.
        Analysis of right ventricular function during bypass of the left side of the
        heart by afterload alterations in both normal and falling hearts. J Thorac
        Cardiovasc Surg 1996;111:1092-102

[9]   Chow E, Farrar DJ. Effects of left ventricular pressure reductions on
        right ventricular systolic performance. Am J Physiol 1989;257:H1878-
        1885

[10]   Zaffran S, Kelly RG, Meilhac SM. Buckingham ME, Brown NA. Right
        ventricular myocardium derives from the anterior heart field. Circ Res
        2004;95:261-268

[11]   Smith SH, Kramer MF, Reis I, Bishop SP, Ingwall JS. Regional changes
        in creatine kinase and myocyte size in hypertensive and nonhypertensive
        cardiac hypertrophy. Circ Res 1990;67:1334-44

[12]   Singh S, White FC, Bloor CM. Myocardial morphometric characteristics
        in swine. Circ Res 1981;49:434-41

[13]   Kusachi S, Nishiyama O, Yasuhara K, Saito D, Haraoka S, Nagashima
        H. Right and left ventricular oxygen metabolism in open-chest dogs. An
        J Physiol 1982;243:H761-6

[14]   Brooks WW, Bing OH, Blaustein AS, Allen PD. Comparison of
        contractile state and myosin isozymes of rat right and left ventricular
        myocardium. J Moll Cell Cardiol 1987;19:433-40

[15]   Sato S, Achrof M, Milliard R. Connective tissue change in early
        ischemia of porcine myocardium, J Moll Cell Cardiol 1983;15:261-69

[16]   Shroff S, Janicki J, Weber K. Left ventricular systolic dynamics in the
        term of its chamber mechanical properties. Am J Physiol
        1983;245:H110-24

[17] Grant RP, Downey FM, Mac Mahon H. The architecture of the right ventricular outflow tract in the normal heart and in the presence of ventricular septal defects. Circulation 1961;24:223

[18] Sarnoff SJ, Berglund E. Ventricular function. I. Starling's law of the heart studied by means of simultaneous right and left ventricular function curves in the dog. Circulation 1954;9:706-718

[19] Starr I, Jeffers WA, Meade RH. The absence of conspicuous increments of venous pressure after severe damage to the right ventricle of the dog, with a discussion of the relation between clinical congestive failure and heart disease. Am Heart J 1943;26:291

[20] Kagan A. Dynamic responses of the right ventricle following extensive damage by cauterization. Circulation 1958;1:724

[21] Suga H, Sagawa K, Shoukas AA. Load independence of the instantaneous pressure-volume ratio of the canine left ventricle and effects of epinephrine and heart rate on the ratio. Cir Res 1973;32:314

[22] Baan J, van der Velde ET, de Bruin HG, Smeenk GJ, Koops J, van Dijk AD, et al. Continuous measurement of left ventricular volume in animals and humans by conductance catheter. Circulation 1984;70:812-23

[23] Maughan WL, Shoukas AA, Sagawa K, Weisfeldt ML. Instantaneous pressure-volume relationship of the canine right ventricle. Circ Res 1979;44:309

[24] Feneley MP, Elbeery JR, Gaynor JW, Gall SA Jr, Davis JW, Rankin JS. Ellipsoidal shell subtraction model of right ventricular volume: Comparison with regional free wall dimensions as indexes of right ventricular function. Circ Res 1990;67:1427-36

[25] Morris JJ, Pellom GL, Hamm DP, Everson CT, Wechsler AS. Dynamic right ventricular dimension. J Thorac Cardiovasc Surg 1986;91:879-887

[26] Dyke CM, Brunsting LA, Salter DR, Murphy CE, Abd-Dlfattah A, Wechsler AS. Preload dependence of right ventricular blood flow: I. The normal right ventricle. Ann Thorac Surg 1987;43:478-483

[27] Stein PD, Sabbah HN, Marzilli M, Anbe DT. Effect of chronic pressure overload on the maximal rate of pressure fall of the right ventricle. Chest 1980;78:10-15

[28] Sabbah HN, Stein PD. Negative diastolic pressure in the intact canine right ventricle: evidence of diastolic suction. Circ Res 1981;49:108-113

[29] Omoto T, Tanabe H, LaRia PJ, Guererro J, Vlahakes GJ. Right ventricular performance during left ventricular unloading conditions: the contribution of the right ventricular free wall. Thorac Cardiovasc Surg 2002;50:16-20

[30] Santamore WP, Dell'Italia. Ventricular interdependence: significant left ventricular contributions to right ventricular systolic function. Prog Cardiovasc Dis 1998;40:289-308

[31] Maughan WI, Sunagawa K, Sagawa K. Ventricular systolic interdependence: volume elastance model in isolated hearts. Am J Physiol 1987;253:H1382-H1390

[32] Bove AA, Santamore WP. Ventricular interdependence. Prog Cardiovasc Dis 1981;23:365-88

[33] Yamaguchi S, Tsuiki K, Miyawaki H, et al. Effect of left ventricular volume on right ventricular end-systolic pressure-volume relation: resetting of regional preload in right ventricular free wall. Circ Res 1989;65:623-31

[34] Woodard JC, Chow E, Farrar DJ. Isolated ventricular systolic interaction during transient reductions in left ventricular pressure. Circ Res 1992;70:944-951

[35] Feneley MP, Gavaghan TP, Baron DW, Branson JA, Roy PR, Morgan JJ. Contributions of left ventricular contraction to the generation of right ventricular systolic pressure in the human heart. Circulation1985;71:473-80

[36] Karunannithi MK, Michiewicz J, Young JA, Feneley MP. Effect of acutely increased left ventricular afterload on work output from the right ventricle in conscious dogs. J Thorac Cardiovasc Surg 2001;121:116-24

[37] Damiano RJ Jr, La Follette P Jr, Cox JL, et al. Significant left ventricular contribution to right ventricular systolic function. Am J Physiol 1991;261:1514-1524

[38] Yamaguchi S, Li KS, Harasawa H, et al. The left ventricle affects the duration of right ventricular ejection. Cardiovasc Res 1993;27:211-215

[39] Santamore WP, Dell'Italia LJ. Ventricular interdependence: significant left ventricular contributions to right ventricular systolic function. Prog Cardiovasc Dis 1998;40:289-308

[40] Kitano M, Nishimura K, Hee PC, Okamoto Y, Ban T. J Thorac Cardiovasc Surg 1994;104:796-803

[41] Vlahakes GJ, Turley K, Hoffman JI. The pathophysiology of failure in acute right ventricular hypertension: hemodynamic and biochemical correlations. Circulation 1981;63:87-95

[42] Murray PA, Baig H, Fishbein MC, Vatner SF. Effects of experimental right ventricular hypertrophy on myocardial blood flow in conscious dogs. J Clin Invest 1979;64:421-427

[43] Fixler DE, Monroe GA, Wheeler JM. Effects of acute right ventricular systolic hypertension on regional myocardial blood flow in anesthetized dogs. Am Heart J 1973;93:210-215

[44] Gold FL, Bache RJ. Transmural right ventricular blood flow during acute pulmonary artery hypertension in the sedated dog. Circ Res 1982;51:196-204

[45] Brooks H, Kik ES, Vokonas PS, Urschel CW, Sonnenblick EH. Performance of the right vetricle under stress: relation to right coronary flow. J Clin Invest 1971;50:2176-2183

[46] Fourier PR, Coetzee AR, Bollinger CT. Pulmonary artery compliance: its role in right ventricular-arterial coulpling. Cardiovasc Res 1992;26:839-844

[47] Puleur H, Lefevre J, van Eyll C, Jaumin PM, Charlier AA. Significance of pulmonary input impedence in right ventricular performance. Cardiovasc Res 1978;12:617-629

[48] Chow E, Farrar DJ. Effects of left ventricular pressure reductions on right ventricular systolic performance. Am J Physiol 1989;257:H1878-1885

[49] Buckberg GD. Endothelial and myocardial stunning. J Thorac Cardiovasc Surg 2000;120:640-641

In: Congestive Heart Failure...   ISBN: 978-1-60876-677-2
Editors: J. E. García et al. pp. 153-162   © 2010 Nova Science Publishers, Inc.

Chapter 7

PLASMA BRAIN NATRIURETIC PEPTIDE – AN INDEPENDENT PREDICTOR OF MORTALITY AND REHOSPITALIZATION IN CONGESTIVE HEART FAILURE – A META-ANALYSIS[*]

Dragos Vesbianu, Carmen Vesbianu, Paul Bernstein and Ruth Kouides

ABSTRACT

Background

CHF is one of the most important cardiac disorders in the US with a high incidence and prevalence as well as increased number of hospitalizations, deaths and, subsequently, increased health care costs.

Design

Meta-analysis of studies assessing BNP as a prognostic indicator.

---

[*] A version of this chapter was also published in World Heart Journal, Volume1, Issue 4, edited by Franz Halberg and R.B. Singh, Nova Science Publishers. It was submitted for appropriate modifications in an effort to encourage wider dissemination of research.

Methods

Our objective is to determine if discharge BNP is an independent predictor of mortality and rehospitalization in patients admitted with CHF exacerbation. Our personal archives, MEDLINE, and reference lists of retrieved articles were searched. Two reviewers checked the list of abstracts and then the full papers for eligible studies and extracted data independently. We have started our search with 954 articles out of which 82 were selected for more detailed review. Only five studies met the eligibility criteria for the final meta-analysis. Our inclusion criteria were: age more than 18 years, CHF diagnosed by Framingham or echo criteria, BNP assessment in the 24 hour period prior to discharge and a minimum follow up period of one month. The outcomes assessed were all cause mortality and rehospitalization. Only observational, prospective cohort studies published in English language were included. We excluded all randomized control trials (as different treatment of different groups will introduce an additional bias), case series, case reports, case control studies, as well as studies that did not indicate clear clinical end points. The quality of the studies was assessed using the QUADAS (Quality Assessment of Diagnostic Accuracy Studies) score. Statistical analyses were performed using the fixed effects model calculated with Stats Direct and results were expressed as relative risks (RR). Receiver Operating Characteristics (ROC) curves were prepared using Dr. ROC software. We have used the I square test to appreciate the heterogeneity of the combined studies.

Results

The RR of death or rehospitalization for the three BNP cutoffs used 250, 350 and 500 pg/ml were 3.87, 4.66 and 5.73 respectively. For the 250 and 350 BNP cutoffs the Area Under the Curve (AUC) was 0.82 and 0.80.

Conclusion

BNP level at discharge is a strong independent predictor of early readmission or death in patients hospitalized with CHF exacerbation. Prior to discharging those patients health care providers should not only assess for clinical stability but also for circulatory stability by checking discharge BNP.

INTRODUCTION

The clinical assessment of congestive heart failure (CHF) is notoriously difficult. It is hard to determine which patients have heart failure and, once the diagnosis is established, to predict which patients are at risk of death or rehospitalization [1].

If we believe in one of the axioms of epidemiology, that disease and death are not chance-determined events, then there must be as yet unidentified characteristics of the patients or interventions that determine the differences in outcome [2].

Brain Natriuretic Peptide (BNP) is a member of the natriuretic peptide family synthesized mainly in the ventricles and secreted in response to myocardial tension or increased intravascular volume. BNP and the amino-terminal fragment of its molecule, N-terminal proBNP (NT-proBNP) have been shown to be independent predictors for mortality and cardiac composite endpoints for populations at risk for coronary artery disease (CAD), diagnosed CAD, and diagnosed HF [3].

Despite many assessments in the literature, the exact relationship between BNP and the prognosis in CHF remains ambiguous. This ambiguity results mainly from the broad range of studies and study designs addressing this topic.

It is well known that heart failure is a syndrome that carries a bad prognosis. Hospitalization is common and rehospitalization rate is high, factors which influence the cost of care [4].

We anticipate that finding a good prognostic indicator for these outcomes will have a major impact on heath care costs of this disease. Hence the objective of this review is to determine if discharge BNP at the time of CHF exacerbation is an independent prognostic factor for mortality or short term rehospitalization.

MATERIAL AND METHODS

Design

We conducted a literature review to estimate the prognostic value of BNP in patients admitted with CHF exacerbation. Only studies that looked at adult patients hospitalized for CHF exacerbation, diagnosed using Framingham [5] or echo criteria were included in the final meta-analysis. Other inclusion criteria were assessing BNP in the 24 hour period prior to discharge and a minimum follow up period of one month. The outcomes assessed were all cause mortality and rehospitalization. Only observational, prospective cohort studies published in English language were included. We excluded all randomized control trials, case series, case reports, case control studies, as well as studies that did not indicate clear clinical end points.

Literature Search

The search for the relevant articles was conducted by three people (the two reviewers and the librarian) using Medline. References from review articles as well as our personal archives were used to find more articles. The time frame was 1989, first year a BNP assay was reported to 2008. We used 5 MeSH terms for BNP and 8 MeSH terms for heart failure. Two different reviewers (DV and CV) evaluated the studies. Conflicts regarding inclusion of the studies were solved by consensus or by the intervention of a third reviewer (RK).

Validity Assessment

The two reviewers independently assessed the methodological quality of prognostic accuracy of each study included in the final analysis using the QUADAS criteria [6]. A quality score based on those criteria was given to each of the studies. We looked at the inclusion criteria, study design, length and completeness of follow up, as well as the blinding of the investigators to the index test or reference standard results.

Data Abstraction

We extracted data on BNP cutoff, the method of measuring BNP, the outcomes assessed, number of events, length of follow up, the number of patients, mean ejection fraction, clinical setting, and study type. The reviewers extracted data independently.

Analysis

Statistical analyses were performed using the fixed effects model calculated with Stats Direct and the results were expressed as relative risks. For the summary ROC curves, AUC as well as for calculating I square to estimate the heterogeneity, we used dr.-ROC software.

RESULTS

We found 926 studies after the MEDLINE search, and we added 28 studies from our personal files and reference lists. After careful evaluation of the titles and abstracts we identified 82 articles for more detailed review. The main reasons for exclusion of the studies were, BNP used to evaluate the response to therapy, the use of NT-proBNP, or usage of BNP as a diagnostic tool. After reviewing the full text of the 82 articles, 77 were excluded mainly for assessing different outcomes, following outpatients only, or no mention of the discharge BNP (Figure 1).

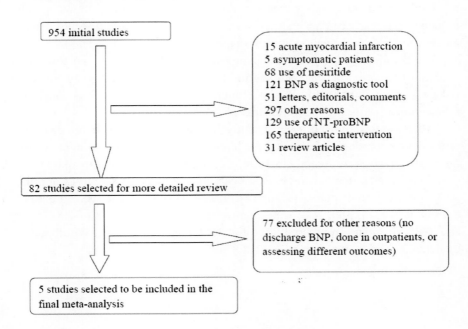

Figure 1. Search strategy

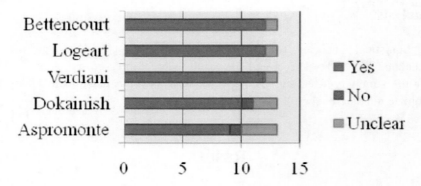

Figure 2. QUADAS criteria per each study

The 5 studies that were included [7, 8, 9, 10, 11] in the final analysis had a total of 607 patients with sample sizes ranging from 50 to 202. The follow up was between 1 and 18 months. The BNP cutoffs used were from 200 to 1170 (Table 1).

The QUADAS score was calculated for each study. Each study receives one point for each quality criterion met. If a study does not satisfy a criterion or if this is not reported it receives zero points. By adding all the points together each study can have a maximum score of 13 points that would denote an ideal study from a methodological quality standpoint. (Figure 2).

We combined the studies depending on their BNP cutoffs. To show the amount of variation between studies and to estimate the overall result (relative risk) we have done a forest plot (Figure 3). Our outcome was death or rehospitalization during the follow up.

All 5 studies showed a consistently increased relative risk for death or rehospitalization during follow up for higher BNP. It is also very evident that the relative risks were steadily increasing as the BNP cutoff used increases.

To appreciate the accuracy we calculated summary ROC curves and the AUC for each BNP cutoff (Figure 4). The ROC curves for the three BNP cutoffs used (225, 350, 500) were relatively similar with AUCs of 0.82, 0.81 and 0.84. I square was used to estimate the heterogeneity. We found a moderate to high heterogeneity.

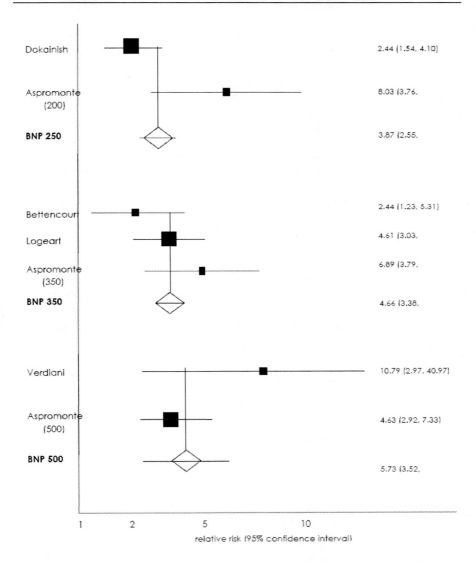

Figure 3. Relative risk meta-analysis plot (fixed effect) for all three BNP cutoffs.

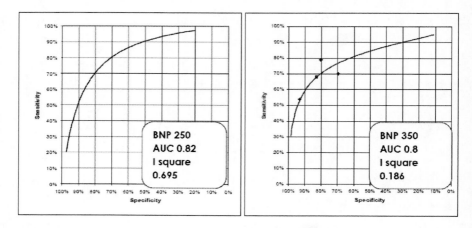

Figure 4. ROC curves, AUCs and I square for two of the BNP cutoffs.

There are several factors that seemed to be fair predictors of mortality. Older age, comorbidities such as diabetes mellitus or renal dysfunction, higher NYHA class, lower ejection fraction, hyponatremia, lower body mass index, lower blood pressure, and lower quality life scores. However none of these is a strong predictor [11].

DISCUSSION

The cost of CHF hospitalization is very high and numerous attempts were done to determine which factors can increase hospital readmission or mortality.

It is difficult to point to the exact BNP cutoff that we should aim for. Health care providers should not only assess the patients' clinical stability but also their circulatory stability by checking BNP prior to discharge. Doing so we may be able to identify those patients who have a high risk of rehospitalization or death and either postpone their discharge or arrange for a closer follow up as outpatients.

We have conducted a high-quality and reproducible review there are a few limitations. Although we have started with a large number of trials we had to limit our final analysis to only five. Because the BNP cutoffs used were so heterogeneous we had to split them in more subgroups. Taking into consideration only studies that were published in English, there is a potential for publication bias. It is possible that small studies or studies that did not come up with positive results were never published.

Our meta-analysis of the various published data showed that discharge BNP is an excellent prognostic indicator for hospital readmission or death in patients hospitalized for heart failure exacerbation.

Table 1. Baseline characteristics

Study name	No of patients	BNP cutoffs	Follow up (months)	Mean age	Mean EF %	Outcome	No of events
Aspromonte	145	200,250,350 500	6	72	42	Death or readmission	41
Dokainish	110	250	18	59	40	Death or readmission	54
Bettencourt	50	321	6	71	NR	Death or readmission	20
Logeart	202	350, 700	6	70	34	Death or readmission	86
Verdiani	100	506, 696, 789, 1170	1	78	38	Death or readmission	17

REFERENCES

[1]   Doust, JA; Pietrzak, E. How well does B-type natriuretic peptide predict death and cardiac events in patients with heart failure: systematic review. *BMJ,* 2005, 330.

[2]   Bettencourt, P; Frioes, F; Azevedo, A. Prognostic information provided by serial measurements of brain natriuretic peptide in heart failure. *International Journal of Cardiology,* 2004, 93, 45-48.

[3]   Testing for BNP and NT-proBNP in the diagnosis and prognosis of heart failure. AHRQ (Agency for Healthcare Research and Quality). Publication No. 06-E014, Sept. 2006.

[4]   Linee, A. Health care costs of heart failure: results from a randomized study of patient education. *European Journal of Heart Failure,* 2000, 2, 291-297.

[5]   McKee, PA; Castelli, WP; McNamara, PM; Kannel, WB. The natural history of CHF. The Framingham study. *N Engl J Med,* 1971, 285, 1442-1446.

[6]   Hatjimihail, A. Quality of diagnostic accuracy studies: the development, use and evaluation of QUADAS. *Evid. Based Med.*, 2006, 11, 189.

[7]   Aspromonte, N; Feola, M; Milli, M. prognostic role of B-type natriuretic peptide in patients with diabetes and acute decompensated heart failure. *Diabetic Medicine,* 2007, 24, 124-130.

[8]   Dokainish, H; Zoghbi, WA; Ambriz, E. Comparative cost-effectiveness of B-type natriuretic peptide and echocardiography for predicting outcome in patients with congestive heart failure. *Am. J. Cardiol,* 2005, 97, 400-403.

[9]   Bettencourt, P; Ferreira, S; Azevedo, A. Preliminary data on the potential usefulness of B-type natriuretic petide levels in predicting outcome after hospital discharge in patients with heart failure. *Am J Med.,* 2002, 113, 215-219.

[10]   Logeart, D; Thabut, G; Jourdain, P. Pre-discharge B-type natriuretic peptide assay for identifying patients at risk of re-admission after decompensated heart failure. *J. Am. Coll Cardiol.,* 2004, 43, 635-41.

[11]   Verdiani, V; Nozzoli, C; Bacci, F. Pre-discharge B-type natriuretic peptide predicts early reccurence of decompensated heart failure in patients admitted to a general medical unit. *Eur J. Heart Failure,* 2005, 7, 566-571.

In: Congestive Heart Failure…   ISBN: 978-1-60876-677-2
Editors: J. E. García et al. pp. 163-207   © 2010 Nova Science Publishers, Inc.

Chapter 8

CONGESTIVE HEART FAILURE: DIFFERENT NON-INVASIVE DIAGNOSIS TECHNIQUES[*]

Abdulnasir Hossen and Bader Al Ghunaimi
Department of Electrical and Computer Engineering
College of Engineering
Sultan Qaboos University
P.O.Box 33 Al-Khod, 123 Oman

ABSTRACT

Heart rate variability is analyzed in time-domain or in frequency-domain. Three different novel non-invasive techniques for analysis of heart rate variability (R-R interval (RRI)) for the screening of patients with Congestive Heart Failure (CHF) are investigated. The first method, which is a time-domain method, is based on the Statistical Signal Characterization (SSC) of the analytical signal that is generated using Hilbert transformation of the RRI data. The four SSC parameters are: amplitude mean, period mean, amplitude deviation and period deviation. These parameters and their maximum and minimum values are determined over sliding segments of 300-samples, 32-samples and 16-

---

[*] A version of this chapter was also published in Artificial Intelligence: New Research, edited by R.B. Bernstein and W.N. Curtis, Nova Science Publishers. It was submitted for appropriate modifications in an effort to encourage wider dissemination of research.

samples for both the instantaneous amplitudes and the instantaneous frequencies derived from the analytical signal of the RRI data. Data used in this work are drawn from MIT database. The trial data used for estimating of the classification factor consists of 15 CHF (patient) subjects and 18 Normal Sinus Rhythm (NSR) or simply normal subjects. The performance of the algorithm is then evaluated on test data set consists of 17 CHF subjects and 53 NSR subjects. This new technique correctly classifies 31/33 of trial data and 65/70 of test data

The second and third techniques, which are frequency-domain methods, are based on the soft-decision wavelet-decomposition algorithm for estimating an approximate power spectral density (PSD) of (RRI) of ECG data for screening of congestive heart failure (CHF) from normal subjects. In the second method, the ratio of the power in the low-frequency (LF) band to the power in the high-frequency (HF) band of the RRI signal is used as the classification factor. Results are shown for 9 different wavelets filters. This new technique shows a classification efficiency of 93.93% on trial data and 88.57% on test data. An FFT-based frequency domain screening technique is also implemented and included in this chapter for the purpose of comparison with the wavelet-based technique. The FFT-based technique shows an efficiency of classification of 93.93% on trial data and 81.42% on test data.

In the third technique, which is a pattern recognition technique, two standard patterns of the base-2 logarithmic values of the reciprocal of the approximate PSD of sub-bands resulted from wavelet decomposition of RRI data of CHF patients and normal subjects are derived by averaging all corresponding values of all sub-bands of 12 CHF data and 12 normal subjects in the trial set. The computed pattern of each data under test is then compared band-by-band with both standard patterns of CHF and normal subjects to find the closest pattern. This new simple technique results in 90% identification accuracy by applying it on the test data.

Keywords: Non-Invasive Diagnosis, Congestive Heart Failure, Heart Rate Variability, Time-Domain Analysis, Statistical Signal Characterization, Frequency-Domain Analysis, Wavelet Decomposition and FFT, Pattern Recognition.

1. INTRODUCTION

1.1. Heart Failure

Heart failure is a common condition that usually develops slowly as the heart muscle weakens and needs to work harder to maintain a normal organ blood supply. Heart failure develops following death of heart muscle cells caused by myocardial infarction, pressure overload due to untreated high blood pressure, or due to abnormality of one of the heart valves [1]. A more advanced stage of the disease, commonly referred to as Congestive Heart Failure (CHF), refers to failure of both left and right ventricles causing fluid to accumulate in the lungs, lower limbs, liver and sometimes the abdominal cavity.

According to the New York Heart Association (NYHA), heart failure is classified into four classes:

Class I (Mild), Symptoms with more than ordinary activity.
Class II (Mild), Symptoms with ordinary activity.
Class III (Moderate), Symptoms with minimal activity.
Class IV (Severe), Symptoms at rest.

Physicians often order a number of tests when exploring a possible diagnosis of heart failure. The most important of these is the Echocardiogram, which is a noninvasive technique using ultrasound to image the heart as it is beating in real time. It provides accurate measures of ventricular size, degree of contractility and valve function, as well the amount and direction of blood flow through heart chambers. It can thus determine the degree of failure, some of the causes and whether it is on the left ventricle, the right ventricle, or both [1]. The information from the Echocardiography is also used for calculating the ejection fraction (EF), which is the percent of the blood pumped out during each heartbeat. EF is a simple important measure for determining the severity of heart failure. People with a healthy heart usually have an EF of 50 percent or greater. Most people with heart failure, but not all, have an EF of 40 percent or less [1].

1.2. Heart Rate Variability (HRV)

HRV is referred to as the beat-to-beat variation in heart rate. Instantaneous heart rate is measured as the time in seconds between peaks of two consecutive R waves of the ECG signal. This time is referred to as the RRI. The variation of heart rate accompanies the variation of several physiological activities such as breathing, thermoregulation and blood pressure changes. HRV is a result of continuous alteration of the autonomic neural regulation of the heart i.e. the variation of the balance between sympathetic and parasympathetic neural activity. The increase of sympathetic tone or decrease of parasympathetic activity will increase heart rate [2].

HRV analysis serves as a marker for cardiovascular disease because cardiac dysfunction is often manifested by systematic changes in the variability of the RRI sequence relative to that of normal subjects. Several HRV abnormalities have been described in patients with CHF. It has been shown that patients with CHF have decreased HRV, which can be used as a risk factor for sudden cardiac arrest [3].

HRV analysis involves the manipulation of the RRI data either in time domain or in frequency domain. The analysis either processes the entire RRI data at once or processes subsequent segments (e.g. 5-minutes) of the RRI data.

Several time domain and frequency domain measures of HRV had been examined for discriminating Normal Sinus Rhythm (NSR) and CHF subjects at different window lengths [4]. It is mentioned that the normal subjects exhibit greater fluctuation at scale window between 16 and 32 samples than those afflicted with heart failure. It was possible to completely discriminate between the two groups of 15 CHF and 12 NSR subjects that are part of the trial data in this study.

HRV has shown to be reduced in CHF and in children with congenital heart disease [5]. Some time domain measures, like the standard deviation of the normal RR interval (SDNN), the standard deviation of the averages of NN intervals in all 5-minutes segments (SDANN) and the number of pairs of adjacent NN intervals differing by more than 50 msec divided by the total number of all NN intervals (pNN50), correlated significantly with severity (EF) of heart failure. Highest discrimination power (accuracy of 93.2%) of SDNN measure was also revealed by [6] in separating 52 NSR subjects and 22 CHF patients using linear discrimination analysis. Moreover, it is found in [7] that the pNN less than 50 msec consistently provided better separation between 72 health subjects and 42 CHF patients. Enhanced separation was obtained by using pNN threshold as low as 20 msec or less.

Frequency-domain analysis approaches use one of the signal transformations such as FFT, STFT and wavelet transform to estimate the power spectral density of the RRI data. The frequency spectrum of the RRI data is divided into three main bands [2]:

The very low-frequency band (VLF): $f \in (0.0033 - 0.04)\ Hz$.
The low-frequency band (LF): $f \in (0.04 - 0.15)\ Hz$.
The high-frequency band (HF): $f \in (0.15 - 0.4)\ Hz$

This work concentrates on discriminating patients with CHF from NSR subjects using three screening algorithms. The first one is a time domain analysis of RRI data, and based on the *Statistical Signal Characterization* (SSC) of the analytical signal that is generated using Hilbert transformation (HT) of the RRI data. Four SSC parameters: amplitude mean, period mean, amplitude deviation and period deviation, and their maximum and minimum values are found over a 300-samples, 32-samples and 16-samples sliding window of the analytical signal [8]. Previous implementation of SSC technique for screening obstructive sleep apnea (OSA) patients from normal subjects resulted in screening accuracy above 90% [9].

The second algorithm is a frequency domain analysis, and based on soft estimation of power entropy of the wavelet-decomposed sub-bands of RRI data [10]. This algorithm was investigated in [11] for screening of OSA patients from normal controls using power entropy ratio of the LF/VLF bands. The algorithm proved its applicability on raw-data and resulted in perfect classification results of 100%. In [12 and [13], screening of OSA and normal controls was achieved by estimating the PSD using the soft-decision algorithm on decomposed sub-bands. The same method was also used to screen patients with CHF using power spectral ratios LF/HF and VLF/LF as screening parameters on MIT trial data [14].

The estimation of PSD using wavelet decompositions instead of sub-band decomposition was introduced in [15].

The third algorithm, which is also a frequency domain algorithm, is a pattern recognition algorithm derived mainly from the second algorithm. The whole PSD spectrum is used for the purpose of comparing the spectrum of the data under test with two standard plots derived from CHF and normal trial data to find the closest pattern. A screening accuracy of 90% is obtained on 70 MIT test data.

2. MATERIAL

2.1. Data

The CHF records and NSR records were drawn from MIT[1] database [16]. Two groups of CHF and NSR records are used as described below.

2.2.1. Trial Group

This group contains 15 CHF and 18 NSR records from MIT-BIH database [16]. These records are used to setup the classification algorithm, which is then applied to the test records. The subjects of CHF are 11 men with age between 22 and 71 years, and 4 women with age between 54 and 63 years; all with CHF (NYHA class 3-4). The duration of each record is about 20 hours. The subjects were part of a larger study group receiving conventional medical therapy *prior* to receiving the oral inotropic agent, milrinone. The subjects of the NSR records are 5 men, with age between 26 and 45 years, and 13 women with age between 20 and 50 years. The subjects were found to have no significant arrhythmias.

2.1.2. Test Group

This group contains 17 CHF and 53 NSR recordings that are used to test the performance of the classification algorithm. The CHF subjects are selected from a larger set that contains 29 long-term recordings. The selected 17 records have CHF with NYHA class 3, and the remaining 12 records have NYHA class 1 and 2, and therefore have been excluded from the study. The subjects for the selected records are 8 men, aged 39 to 68, and 2 women aged 38 and 59; gender is unknown for the 7 remaining records, but aged between 35 and 64 years. The NSR data of this group contains 53 long-term (about 24 hours) RRI records. The subjects are 30 men aged 28.5 to 76, and 24 women aged 58 to 73.

The RRI data, for the trial and test groups, are generated from the annotation file, which is associated with each record, using WFDB software [17].

---

[1] MIT: Massachusetts Institute of Technology

2.2. Pre-processing of RRI Data

The RRI data could contain false intervals, missed intervals and/or ectopic intervals that accumulate during RRI generation process; this is because the original ECG is normally exposed to different types of physiological and environmental disturbances, furthermore due to the imperfect performance of QRS detectors that could miss normal peaks or detect false or ectopic beats [18, 19]. Large errors induced by missing values, outliers, non-stationarity and irregular inter-sample spacing could influence the accuracy of any spectral or statistical analysis.

The processing steps involved in this work are shown in the block-diagram of Figure 1. The CHF and NSR records are available in different lengths. Therefore all records are truncated to the minimum record length, which are 75106 samples before starting any processing. The first step in RRI data processing is to bound the RRI values between two limits: 0.4 Sec and 2 Sec, so that all intervals beyond these limits are rejected [20]. The resultant data are then re-sampled at 1 Hz by linear interpolation to substitute for missing values and to obtain equally spaced RRI data, at one second intervals, which is necessary for time domain and frequency domain analysis [18, 20]. This process also involves the removal of DC component from RRI time series by subtracting the mean value. Hereafter, the RRI refer to the filtered RRI data shown in Figure 1.

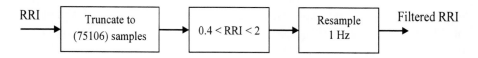

Figure 1. Processing of RRI data.

3. METHODS

This section present theoretical background of the two analysis method: the Statistical signal Characterization and the Soft-Decision Wavelet decomposition, and the Receiver Operating Characteristics which is used for performance evaluation of the two analysis methods.

3.1. Method 1: Statistical Signal Characterization

The analysis steps of SSC algorithm are shown in Figure 2. The SSC is applied to the amplitude (after normalization) and frequency attributes of the RRI data, which are generated by Hilbert transform (HT). The analysis stages are described as follows.

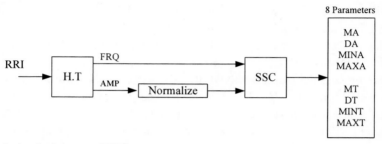

Figure 2. Analysis steps of SSC.

3.1.1. Hilbert Transform (HT)

Hilbert transform is a technique that is used to calculate the instantaneous attributes of a time series. The attributes of a time series are its *amplitude, phase, and frequency*. The result of Hilbert transform is called the *analytical signal,* from which the attributes are to be calculated. The analytical signal has a real part, which is the original signal, and an imaginary part, which is the Hilbert transform. The imaginary part is a 90° phase shifted version of the original signal. The amplitude and phase attributes are the amplitude and phase of the analytical signal [21, 22]. The frequency attribute is the derivative of phase attribute, θ.

$$Amplitude = \sqrt{\operatorname{Re}(x)^2 + \operatorname{Im}(x)^2} \tag{1}$$

$$Frequency = \frac{d\theta}{dt} = rate\ of\ change\ of\ instantaneous\ phase\ (radians) \tag{2}$$

If the time between two consecutive instantaneous phases is constant, the frequency attribute could be regarded as the difference in two successive phases as follows:

$$Frequency = (\theta_{n+1} - \theta_n)/2.\pi\ (Hz); \tag{3}$$

Normalization of the instantaneous amplitude is achieved by dividing the amplitudes values in each data set by its mean value. Normalization is intended to compromise between the variations of different subjects.

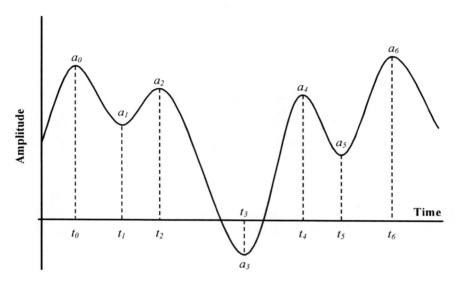

Figure 3. The segments of RRI signal by SSC process.

3.1.2. Statistical Signal Characterization (SSC)

SSC is a statistical method that characterizes a signal by four basic parameters: amplitude mean (M_a), amplitude deviation (D_a), period mean (M_t), and period deviation (D_t), which will be described in the context of this section. SSC concept is simple to interpret, and the parameters are mathematically and computationally simple to calculate.

The input waveform to the SSC process is basically divided into segments; each segment is bounded by two extrema: maxima and minima as in Figure 3 [23]. The segment amplitude (A) and the segment period (T) are defined as:

Segments Amplitude vector, $A_n = |a_n - a_{n-1}|$ (4)

where,

A_n = amplitude of the nth segment,

a_n = waveform amplitude at the concluding extremum of the segment,

a_{n-1} = waveform amplitude at the begining extremum of the segment.

Segments Period vector, $T_n = t_n - t_{n-1}$ (5)

Where,

T_n = period of the nth segment,

t_n = waveform elapsed time at the concluding extremum of the segment,

t_{n-1} = waveform elapsed time at the begining extremum of the segment.

Four SSC parameters could be computed from the amplitude and period vectors of the signal under process. The parameters are the amplitude mean M_a, the period mean M_t, the amplitude mean deviation D_a, and the period mean deviation D_t:

$$M_a = \sum_{i=1}^{N_s} (A_i / N_s)$$ (6)

$$M_t = \sum_{i=1}^{N_s} (T_i / N_s)$$ (7)

$$D_a = \sum_{i=1}^{N_s} (|A_i - M_a|) / N_s$$ (8)

$$D_t = \sum_{i=1}^{N_s} (|T_i - M_t|) / N_s$$ (9)

Where A_i is the amplitude of the ith segment, and T_i is the period of the ith segment and N_s is the total number of segments.

The frequency (FRQ) and amplitude (AMP) attribute signals in Figure 2 are then passed to the SSC process. The SSC process is applied to 3 versions of window length: 300-samples (5-minutes), 32-samples (32 seconds), and 16-samples (16 seconds). The four SSC parameters are calculated for every window that slides by one window length after each SSC process, in other word, for each processed window of the RRI data, there is a single value for each SSC parameter.

In addition to these four SSC parameters, other four parameters are calculated that represent the minimum and maximum values of the segments amplitudes (A) and segments periods (T) within the window under process.

$$MINA = Min(A) \tag{10}$$

$$MAXA = Max(A) \tag{11}$$

$$MINT = Min(T) \tag{12}$$

$$MAXT = Max(T) \tag{13}$$

The 8 SSC parameters are used as promising classifiers of RRI data which will be evaluated for their screening capabilities. The method of classifying the CHF and NSR subjects is based on the number of windows from the total record windows for which an SSC parameter is below certain predefined threshold (SSCTHR). If the ratio of the minutes is below a certain ratio threshold (ROCTHR), the record is classified as CHF otherwise it is a NSR record. Therefore, two threshold values are required to be set for each SSC parameter; one for the SSC parameter itself (SSCTHR) and the other for the ratio of minutes (ROCTHR). The selection of optimal threshold values is accomplished with the help of Receiver-Operating-Characteristic (ROC) analysis as described in the section 3.3.

3.2. Method 2: Soft-Decision Wavelet Decomposition

3.2.1. Wavelet-decomposition of RRI signal

The block-diagram of the wavelet decomposition is shown in Figure 4. The wavelet decomposition starts by filtering the input RRI signal $x(n)$ of length-N by low-pass (LPF) and high-pass (HPF) filters and then down-sampled by a factor of 2 to produce both the "approximation" $a(n)$ and the "details" $d(n)$. Assuming haar-filters are used, then $a(n)$ and $d(n)$ can be obtained by:

$$a(n) = \frac{1}{\sqrt{2}}[x(2n) + x(2n+1)]$$

$$d(n) = \frac{1}{\sqrt{2}}[x(2n) - x(2n+1)] \qquad (14)$$

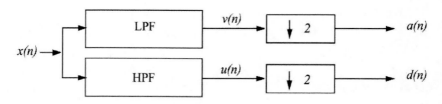

Figure 4. Single wavelet decomposition stage.

If it is known that the energy is concentrated in one of the bands, a process could be applied in that band and stopped in the other resulting in reduced complexity and processing time. The decomposed bands could also be decomposed further and further into high frequency and low frequency sub-bands using the same filters. The process of selecting one decomposition path out of the full decomposition is called hard decision algorithm [24]. The band selection is established by the energy comparison between the low- and high-frequency subsequences after the down sampling $a(n)$ and $d(n)$:

$$B = \sum_{n=0}^{\frac{N}{2}-1} (a(n))^2 - (d(n))^2 \qquad (15)$$

According to the sign of B, the decision is taken: If B is positive, the low-frequency band is considered, and if B is negative, the high-frequency band is considered. Since we are not interested in the value of B, but only in its sign, Equation 15 can be simplified to:

$$\text{sgn}(B) = \text{sgn} \sum_{n=0}^{\frac{N}{2}-1} |a(n)| - |d(n)| \qquad (16)$$

Energy comparison and band selection is repeated at each decomposition stage resulting in following one decomposition path and narrowing down the estimate of the dominant frequency range of the original sequence. Given its simplicity, the method of hard decision estimation may not be very reliable in practice because at each stage the approximations to the estimated quantities are crude resulting in a high error probability. A particularly useful modification of the hard decision algorithm is to perform full decomposition in each stage to specified number of times and assign a probability measure that reflects the energy in each decomposed band. This process is called the soft decision algorithm [22] and found useful in estimating an approximate power spectral density (PSD) of the RRI signal as described below.

3.2.2. Estimation of Power Spectral Density

The following procedure is used to estimate the PSD of the decomposed sub-bands [15]:

1.   The wavelet-decompositions are computed with all branches up to a certain stage m to obtain 2^m sub-bands.
2.   All estimator results up to stage m are stored, and a probability measure is assigned to each path (i.e., frequency band) to bear the primary information.
3.   If $J(L)$ is the assigned probability of the input signal being primarily low-pass, the number $J(H) = 1- J(L)$ is the probability that the signal is primarily high-pass. One simple way to make the probability assignments is to use the ratio of the number of positive comparisons between $|a(n)|$ and $|d(n)|$ in Equation (16) to the total number of comparisons for a given stage.
4.   At the following stage, the resulting estimate can be interpreted as the conditional probability of the new input sequence containing primarily low (high) frequency components, given that the previous branch was predominantly low (high)-pass. Using this reasoning and laws of probability, the assignments for the probability measure of the resulting sub-bands should be made equal to the product of the previous branch probability and the conditional probability estimated at a given stage. Figure 5 shows this step of probability assignment for 8 sub-bands.

5. The probabilities $P(B_i)$ derived from the estimator outputs, where i is the index of the band, may be interpreted themselves as a coarse measurement of the PSD: The higher the probability value of any band, the higher is its power-spectral content. For m decomposition stages, 2^m bands are resulted. Each band covers $(0.5/2^m)$ Hz of the RRI spectrum (0-0.5) Hz.

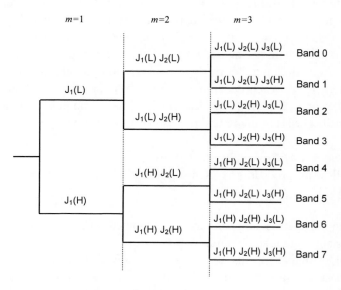

Figure 5. PSD estimation by probability measures.

3.2.3. Implementation on MIT-Trial Data

The soft-decision algorithm is implemented on the MIT-trial data using haar wavelet filters with $m=5$ decomposition stages resulting in 32 frequency bands. The PSD (the probability values) of the 32 bands are obtained for each normal record and CHF record. An average PSD plot is derived for each case (CHF and normal) by averaging the probability values of counterpart bands in each case. The average PSD plots of the 18 normal records and the 15 CHF records are shown in Figure 6.

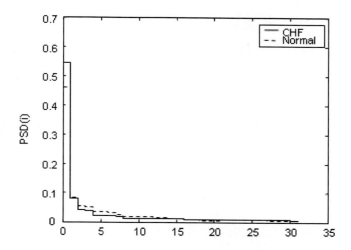

Figure 6. The average PSD plots for the CHF and Normal cases of MIT trial records.

It can be noticed from the plot that normal records have larger values of PSD at the LF band (bands 4 to 10) compared to the CHF records. This is not the case in the HF band (bands 11 to 25) in which the PSD seems to be constant for both. Therefore, the power ratio LF/HF of the PSD could be significant in identification of CHF records from the normal records. The power in the LF band (0.04-0.15) Hz is computed approximately by summing the probability values (PSD) of the bands (4 to 10) as:

$$H_{LF} = \sum_{i=4}^{i=10} P(B_i)$$

(17)

The power in the HF band is computed approximately as:

$$H_{HF} = \sum_{i=11}^{i=25} P(B_i)$$

(18)

A classification factor (CF) can be computed then as:

$$CF = H_{LF} / H_{HF}$$

(19)

3.3. Receiver Operating Characteristics

The performance of a classification algorithm is evaluated by three main metrics: sensitivity, specificity and accuracy as defined below [25]:

$$Sensitivity\ (\%) = \frac{TP}{TP + FN}.100 \tag{20}$$

$$Specificity\ (\%) = \frac{TN}{TN + FP}.100 \tag{21}$$

$$Accuracy\ (\%) = \frac{TP + TN}{TP + FP + TN + FN}.100 \tag{22}$$

While the entities in the above equations are defined as follows and shown in both Table 1 and Figure 7 (All cases above the threshold are assumed positive and all cases below the threshold are assumed negative):

TP (True Positives) is the number of the correctly classified positive cases.
FN (False Negatives) is the number of positive cases that are misclassified as negative.
TN (True Negatives) is the number of the correctly classified negative cases.
FP (False Positives) is the number of negative cases that are misclassified as positive.

Table 1. The Confusion Matrix

		Predicted Class	
		Positive	Negative
Actual	Positive	TP	FN
Class	Negative	FP	TN

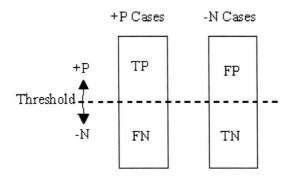

Figure 7. The description of TP, FN, FP and TN in confusion matrix.

Sensitivity represents the ability of a classifier to detect the positive cases, e.g. CHF. Specificity indicates the ability of a classifier to detect negative cases, e.g. normal subjects. Accuracy represents the overall performance of a classifier. It indicates the percentage of correctly classified positive and negative cases from the total cases [25, 26].

The performance of a classifier, which is an SSC parameter or CF in our two algorithms, at different threshold values can be represented graphically using ROC curve. As shown in Figure 8, the ROC space is defined by two coordinates, the x-axis represents the percentage of false positive (FP) cases or (1-specificity) and y-axis represents the sensitivity. ROC curve is produced by spanning the full spectrum of the threshold values and calculating the sensitivity and specificity at each threshold increment. The calculated values are then plotted in the ROC space to represent the performance profile of the classifier. The performance profile of different classifiers could also be plotted in one ROC space to facilitate the comparison between the performances of different classifiers. For orientation, three specific points on the ROC graph should be defined as shown in Figure 8. The bottom left point (0,0) represents the case in which all negative and positive cases are classified as negative. The upper right point (1,1) represents the case in which all positive and negative cases are classified as positive. The upper left point (0,1) is the point of perfect classification (all positive cases are classified as positive and all negative cases are classified as negative). Classifiers that are closer to (0,1) perform better than those located away from this point. The threshold value that produces the highest sensitivity and highest specificity (lowest FP), e.g. produces the closest point to the perfect classification (0,1), is selected to be the optimal threshold value for a given classifier [25, 26, 27].

The results of SSC and Soft Decision algorithms are passed to the ROC analysis. By which the results of the maximum accuracy value are determined and returned.

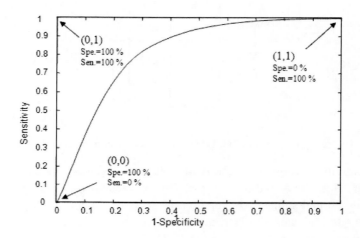

Figure 8. The ROC space and the three extreme points.

3.4. Method 3: Pattern Recognition

The proposed pattern recognition technique is implemented using the following steps [28]:

1. The probability measures are computed for each data of the trial set up to stage m to obtain 2^m probabilities $P(B_i)$, where i is the index of the band. The wavelet filters used are of the type Daubechies (db4). The selection of the wavelet filter is a matter of compromise between the complexity and good filter performances.

2. The logarithmic based-2 values of the reciprocal of the probabilities can be obtained as:

$$I(B_i) = \log_2(\frac{1}{P(B_i)}) \tag{23}$$

A staircase approximation of the values of $I(B_i)$ can be plotted for all bands.

3. An average plot is found by averaging all $I(B_i)$ values of corresponding bands for all 12 CHF data and 12 normal data in the trial set to obtain two standard plots for CHF and normal as in Figure 9 for 32 sub-bands. A clear increase in the values of $I(B_i)$ (clear reduction in the probabilities $P(B_i)$) in the LF region can be noticed in CHF plot compared to that of normal plot.

4. The $I(B_i)$ values for each data under test are found for 32 sub-bands. A classification factor CF is then determined as:

$$CF = \sum_{i=5}^{28} \left(I(B_i) - I_H(B_i) \right)^2 - \sum_{i=5}^{28} \left(I(B_i) - I_N(B_i) \right)^2 \tag{24}$$

Where I_H (B_i) and I_N (B_i) are the standard patterns for CHF and normal respectively.

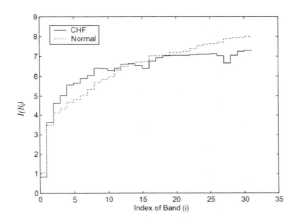

Figure 9. Standard patterns for CHF and normal with 32 sub-bands.

The RRI spectrum in the frequency region (0.0625 Hz – 0.4375 Hz) corresponding to bands 5 to 28 is considered for determining the patterns. The LF and HF regions are used in the recognition, while the VLF and the upper high frequency regions are excluded. Depending on the sign of CF, the

algorithm can decide whether the data is CHF or normal. The data with a
negative CF is considered as normal and the data with a positive CF is a CHF
data.

4. RESULTS AND DISCUSSION

4.1. Results of Method 1: SSC

4.1.1. Results of Trial Data

The results of SSC analysis on amplitude and frequency attributes of trial
data are shown in Figure 10 for window length of 16-samples, 32-samples and
300-samples respectively. In all figures, the x-axis represents the records
index, the y-axis the ratio of windows below SSCTHR threshold.

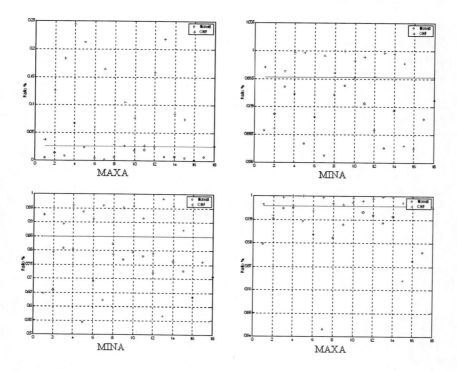

Figure 10 (Continued).

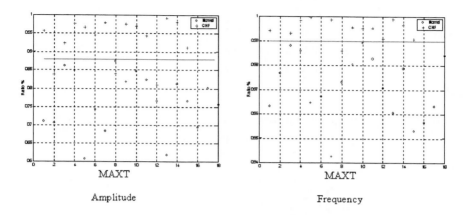

Amplitude   Frequency

Figure 10. Ratio results of amplitude and frequency attributes of trial data at window length of 16-samples.

Tables 2-7 show the specificity, sensitivity and accuracy results, as well as the threshold values at which these results are obtained, for different window lengths and different attributes (amplitude and frequency) of RRI trial data. Out of the eight SSC parameters, the best three parameters, which produced the best accuracies, are selected for the classification algorithm. The selected parameters produced accuracies between 90.9% and 96.97%. These parameters (shown in bold text in the tables) are: MINA, MAXA and MAXT for 16- and 32-samples window, and MT, DT and MAXT for 300-samples window. The selected parameters are the same for amplitude and frequency attributes. In Table 2, MINT also produced accuracy of 90.9% but has been excluded because it was the only case and did not produce the same performance in other window length and attribute.

A voting process is used between the three selected parameters to produce the final classification; a record is classified as CHF if at least two of the three SSC parameters classify (vote) the record as CHF, otherwise it is a NSR record. This is useful in reducing the effect of variance presented in the ratio results as can be perceived from Figure 10. Moreover, it increases the certainty of the classification, especially for those values that are laid close to the ROCTHR. The result of the voting is shown in the last raw of the tables.

As shown in Tables 2-7, the best accuracy, specificity and sensitivity results of the trial data are 96.97%, 100% and 93.3% respectively. These results are obtained on amplitude attribute by MAXA at 16- and 32-samples window, and by MT at 300-samples window. Although the voting process did not produced the maximum accuracy, which obtained by MT and MAXA parameters, the accuracy result is still above 90% with best accuracy, specificity and sensitivity of 93.9%, 100% and 86.7% respectively attained at 300-samples window (Table 4). The maximum specificity of 100%, on trial data, is obtained by most of the SSC parameters, as well as by the voting process.

Table 2. Performance of amplitude attribute of trial data at 16-samples window

	Trial			Thresholds	
SSC	Acc.	Spe.	Sen.	SSC THR	ROC THR
MA	84.85	88.9	80.0	0.328	0.724
DA	81.82	88.9	73.3	0.580	0.637
MINA	**90.91**	**100**	**80.0**	**4.493**	**0.848**
MAXA	**96.97**	**100**	**93.3**	**1.248**	**0.026**
MT	87.9	100	73.3	0.134	0.673
DT	81.8	83.3	80.0	0.0637	0.624
MINT	90.91	83.3	100	1.503	0.959
MAXT	**90.91**	**100**	**80.0**	**1.098**	**0.88**
Voting	**90.91**	**100.0**	**80.0**		

Table 3. Performance of amplitude attribute of trial data at 32-samples window

	Trial			Thresholds	
SSC	Acc.	Spe.	Sen.	SSC THR	ROC THR
MA	84.85	88.9	80.0	0.416	0.885
DA	81.82	94.4	66.7	0.426	0.313
MINA	**90.91**	**100**	**80.0**	**4.422**	**0.685**
MAXA	**96.97**	**100**	**93.3**	**2.127**	**0.825**
MT	87.88	100	73.3	0.134	0.620
DT	78.79	83.3	73.3	0.0468	0.751
MINT	87.88	94.4	80.0	1.503	0.997
MAXT	**93.94**	**100**	**86.7**	**1.424**	**0.963**
Voting	**90.91**	**100.0**	**80.0**		

Table 4. Performance of amplitude attribute of trial data at 300-samples window

	Trial			Thresholds	
SSC	Acc.	Spe.	Sen.	SSC THR	ROC THR
MA	84.85	88.9	80.0	0.364	0.876
DA	81.82	88.9	73.3	0.143	0.495
MINA	72.73	72.2	73.3	0.00064	0.179
MAXA	78.79	83.3	73.3	0.482	0.00953
MT	**96.97**	**100**	**93.3**	**1.878**	**0.714**
DT	**93.94**	**100**	**86.7**	**1.164**	**0.982**
MINT	45.45	0.0	100	1.5	1.000
MAXT	**90.91**	**94.4**	**86.7**	**6.467**	**0.475**
Voting	**93.94**	**100.0**	**86.67**		

In comparison, the frequency attribute of the trial data produced maximum accuracy of 93.9%, with 100% specificity and 86.7% sensitivity, using MINA at 16- and 32- samples window as shown in Tables 5-6. The voting process also produced the same accuracy but at 300-samples window (Table 7).

Table 5. Performance of frequency attribute of trial data at 16-samples window

	Trial			Thresholds	
SSC	Acc.	Spe.	Sen.	SSC THR	ROC THR
MA	69.70	66.7	73.3	0.0463	0.308
DA	69.70	66.7	73.3	0.0763	0.254
MINA	**93.94**	**100**	**86.7**	**5.522**	**0.995**
MAXA	**90.91**	**94.4**	**86.7**	**2.554**	**0.996**
MT	72.73	83.3	60	0.0239	0.505
DT	60.0	50	73.3	0.0202	0.620
MINT	84.85	88.9	80.0	1.503	0.996
MAXT	**90.91**	**100**	**80.0**	**1.103**	**0.990**
Voting	**90.91**	**94.4**	**86.7**		

Table 6. Performance of frequency attribute of trial data at 32-samples window

SSC	Trial			Thresholds	
	Acc.	Spe.	Sen.	SSC THR	ROC THR
MA	72.73	72.3	73.3	0.0436	0.208
DA	72.73	72.3	73.3	0.092	0.214
MINA	**93.94**	**100**	**86.7**	**5.522**	**0.987**
MAXA	**90.91**	**94.4**	**86.7**	**1.768**	**0.911**
MT	72.73	83.3	60.0	0.0235	0.405
DT	57.58	44.4	73.3	0.0159	0.630
MINT	78.79	66.7	93.3	1.005	1.000
MAXT	**90.91**	**100**	**80.0**	**0.929**	**0.990**
Voting	**90.91**	**100**	**80.0**		

Table 7. Performance of frequency attribute of trial data at 300-samples window

SSC	Trial			Thresholds	
	Acc.	Spe.	Sen.	SSC THR	ROC THR
MA	69.70	83.3	53.3	0.041	0.205
DA	66.67	72.2	60.0	0.023	0.180
MINA	54.55	33.3	80	0.0017	0.645
MAXA	66.67	83.3	46.7	0.0576	0.0061
MT	**90.91**	**100**	**80.0**	**1.511**	**0.685**
DT	**87.88**	**88.9**	**86.7**	**0.567**	**0.417**
MINT	45.45	0.0	100	1.500	1.000
MAXT	**90.91**	**100**	**80.0**	**5.418**	**0.878**
Voting	**93.94**	**100**	**86.67**		

4.1.2. Results of Test Data

The results of amplitude and frequency attributes of test data are shown in Figures 11-13 for the three windows lengths. Tables 8-9 show the results of test data using the same parameters and thresholds selected from trial data.

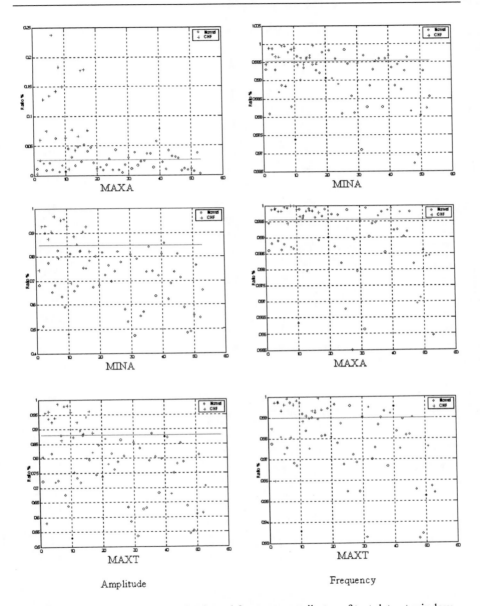

Figure 11. Ratio results of amplitude and frequency attributes of test data at window length of 16-samples.

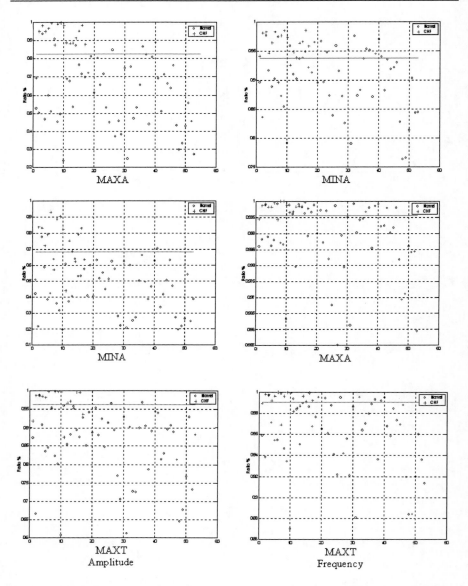

Figure 12. Ratio results of amplitude and frequency attributes of test data at window length of 32-samples.

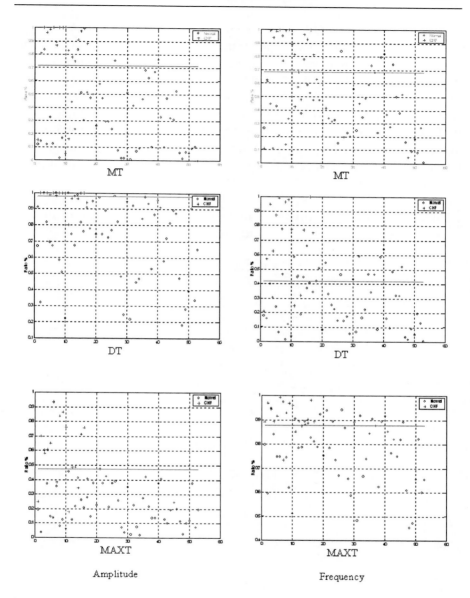

Figure 13. Ratio results of amplitude and frequency attributes of test data at window length of 300-samples.

The maximum accuracy obtained on test data is 92.9% with specificity and sensitivity of 96.2% and 82.4% respectively. This result is obtained by MAXT and the voting process on amplitude attribute at window length of 16-samples (Table 8). Frequency attribute shows lower performance (accuracy below 80%) with best of 77.1% at window length of 300-samples as shown in Table 9. It should be noted that the voting process on amplitude and frequency attributes produced the same maximum accuracy of 93.9% on the trial data, whereas it produced the maximum accuracy of 92.9% only on amplitude attribute of test data, but relatively lower accuracy of 77.1% on frequency attribute of test data.

Table 8. Results of amplitude attribute of test data at different window lengths

	RRI-16-AMP			RRI-32-AMP			RRI-300-AMP		
SSC	Acc.	Spe.	Sen.	Acc.	Spe.	Sen.	Acc.	Spe.	Sen.
MINA	87.14	96.2	58.8	90	96.2	70.6	-	-	-
MAXA	68.57	62.3	88.2	87.1	86.8	88.2	-	-	-
MT	-	-	-	-	-	-	88.57	88.7	88.2
DT	-	-	-	-	-	-	85.71	90.6	70.6
MAXT	92.86	96.2	82.4	88.6	94.3	70.6	91.43	98.1	70.6
Voting	92.86	96.23	82.35	88.6	94.3	70.6	87.14	90.57	76.47

Table 9. Results of frequency attribute of test data at different window lengths

	RRI-16-FRQ			RRI-32-FRQ			RRI-300-FRQ		
SSC	Acc.	Spe.	Sen.	Acc.	Spe.	Sen.	Acc.	Spe.	Sen.
MINA	72.9	73.6	70.6	72.9	73.6	70.6	-	-	-
MAXA	70.0	64.2	88.2	78.6	79.2	88.2	-	-	-
MT	-	-	-	-	-	-	81.4	84.9	70.6
DT	-	-	-	-	-	-	72.9	69.8	82.4
MAXT	72.9	71.7	76.5	74.3	73.6	88.2	74.3	71.7	82.4
Voting	72.9	71.7	76.5	74.3	73.6	88.2	77.14	75.5	82.4

4.1.3. Discussion on SSC results

By observing the performance results of amplitude and frequency attributes of trial data at different window lengths, it is noted that there is no change in the performance of voting process at window length of 16- and 32-samples, but performance improvement observed at 300-samples window. Moreover, some SSC parameters over-perform the others at different window lengths; for example, MINA and MAXA over perform MT and DT at 16- and 32-samples window, and vise versa at 300-samples window. MAXT has almost a stable performance on different attributes and at different windows length in both data groups. It is not significantly affected by the change in window length. Furthermore, all SSC parameters used at different window length have relatively higher specificity (ability to detect the normal records) compared to sensitivity in both trial and test data.

4.1.4. Comparison with Other Studies

Part of our trial data had been investigated in [4], which used the same 15 CHF records but only 12 NSR records compared to 18 records in our study. Accuracy of 100% is achieved in the study at window scales of 16-samples and 32-samples using some individual parameters; no voting between parameters was used. By using a single SSC parameter, MAXA or MT, we could classify 26 out of the 27 records (accuracy of 96.3%) that were used by [4] and 31 out of the 33 records (accuracy of 96.97%) used in this study. However, lower accuracy of 93.4% was obtained when using the voting process. The test data were not used in [4] and therefore these parameters were not tested on test data presented in current study.

The test data in our study was also investigated in [6], which used the same 52 NSR out of 53 records, but 22 CHF (Class 1, 2 and 3). Our study used the 17 class-3 CHF records. The accuracy, specificity and sensitivity of 93.2% (69/74), 98.1% and 81.8% were obtained respectively by [6], which slightly higher than our accuracy of 92.9 % (65/70) but with more CHF records. In addition, the algorithm used was not tested on trial data presented here.

4.2. Results of Method 2: Soft-Decision Wavelet Decomposition

Figure 14 shows the ROC plot for selecting the optimal threshold value for CF results shown in Figure 15. The arrow in the ROC plot indicates the selected threshold and the corresponding sensitivity, specificity and accuracy values. This threshold value is used then to test the performance of the algorithm and the wavelet filter in screening the test data using also db1 filter.

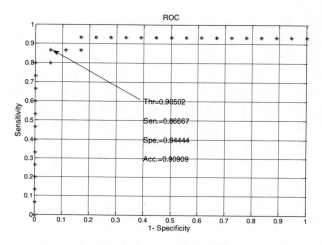

Figure 14. The ROC plot for selecting the optimal threshold value for MIT trial data using db1 wavelet decomposition.

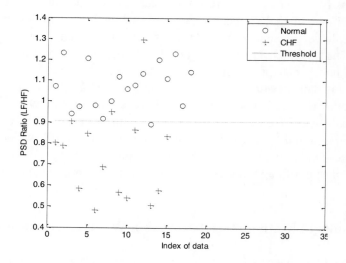

Figure 15. The LF/HF ratio (CF) for MIT RRI trial data using db1 (haar) wavelet decomposition.

Nine wavelet decomposition filters are examined for screening the CHF and normal subjects of test data. The CF threshold values of these filters are setup using the trial data via ROC. The performances of the algorithm using different wavelet filters are then examined on the test data.

Table 10 and Table 11 show the threshold values and the resultant performance on MIT trial and MIT test data respectively. Figure 16 shows the CF plots for MIT test data for selected wavelet filters.

Table 10. The performance of different wavelet decomposition of MIT-trial using (LF/HF)

Wavelet	CF Threshold[a]	Sen. %	Spec. %	Accuracy %
haar	0.905	86.7	94.45	90.9
db2	0.9934	93.3	94.45	93.93
db4	1.007	93.3	94.45	93.93
coif1	1.002	93.3	94.45	93.93
coif3	1.02	93.3	94.45	93.93
coif5	1.017	93.3	94.45	93.93
sym3	1.004	93.3	94.45	93.93
sym4	1.009	93.3	94.45	93.93
Dmey	1.0057	93.3	94.45	93.93

[a] If CF < CF threshold then the record is CHF, otherwise it is a normal record.

Table 11. The performance of different wavelet decomposition of MIT-test using (LF/HF)

Wavelet	CF Threshold[a]	Sen. %	Spec. %	Accuracy %
haar	0.905	82.4	88.7	87.1
db2	0.9934	82.4	90.6	88.6
db4	1.007	82.4	90.6	88.6
coif1	1.002	82.4	88.7	87.1
coif3	1.02	82.4	90.6	88.6
coif5	1.017	82.4	90.6	88.6
sym3	1.004	82.4	90.6	88.6
sym4	1.009	82.4	90.6	88.6
dmey	1.0057	82.4	90.6	88.6

[a] If CF < CF threshold then the record is CHF, otherwise it is a normal record.

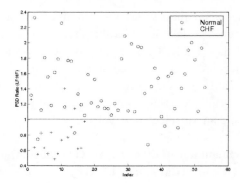

Figure 16. (a) db-4

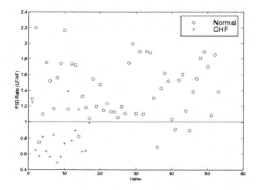

Figure 16. (b) sym3

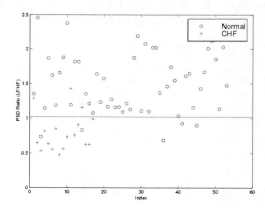

Figure 16. (c) coif-3

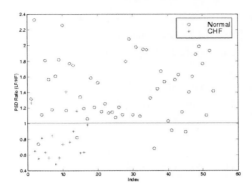

Figure 16. (d) sym-4

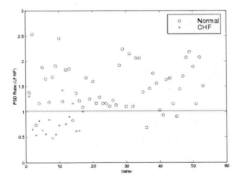

Figure 16. (e) coif-5

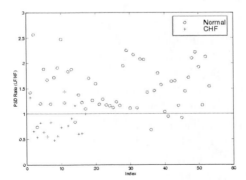

Figure 16.(f) dmey. The LF/HF (CF) plots for MIT test data using different wavelet decomposition filters.

The performance of the algorithm in test data using the different wavelets is almost the same. For further comparison of the screening capability of the 9 wavelets, three different distance metrics [11] are used:

NMSD: Negative Mean Square Distance, which measures the mean square distance of the correct negative outputs (normal) from the threshold and is defined as:

$$NMSD = \sum_i (CF_n(i) - thr)^2 / NP \qquad (25)$$

PMSD: Positive Mean Square Distance, which measures the mean square distance of the correct positive outputs (CHF) from the threshold and is defined as:

$$PMSD = \sum_i (CF_p(i) - thr)^2 / NN \qquad (26)$$

TMSD: Total Mean Square Distance, which measures the mean square distance of all correct outputs (normal and CHF) from the threshold and is defined as:

$$TMSD = \sum_i (CF(i) - thr)^2 / NT \qquad (27)$$

where $CF_n(i)$, $CF_p(i)$ and $CF(i)$ are ratio results for negative (normal), positive (CHF) and all MIT-test records respectively. The NP, NN and NT are the numbers of correct positives, correct negatives and the correct total respectively, and *thr* is the CF threshold value listed in Table 10. Table 12 shows these computed metrics for the 9 different wavelets.

As can be observed in Table 10 and Table 11, a specificity of 94.45% and a sensitivity of 93.33% are obtained by all wavelets filters on MIT trial data except with the haar (db1) filter, with which a specificity of 94.45 and a sensitivity of 86.7% are resulted. The results in Table 11 show almost 88.6% accuracy with 7 wavelet filters on MIT test data. The other two wavelet filters (haar and coif1) result in 87.1% accuracy. It is also shown that the specificity results are higher than the sensitivity results in all filters.

The distance metrics listed in Table 12 show that dmey and coif5 filters have the largest TMSD, NMSD and PMSD. Coif3 filter and sym4 filters are coming in the second level of having higher values of the distance metrics. The haar filter has the lowest values of all metrics.

Table 12. Distance metrics and complexity of different wavelets

Wavelet	TMSD	NMSD	PMSD	Complexity
Haar	0.083	0.0965	0.0392	1.00
db2	0.1864	0.2121	0.098	1.95
db4	0.312	0.368	0.118	3.87
coif1	0.1895	0.2149	0.1042	2.91
coif3	0.3556	0.4258	0.1152	8.54
coif5	0.3943	0.4723	0.127	14.37
sym3	0.269	0.3148	0.113	2.91
sym4	0.310	0.3662	0.1189	3.87
dmey	0.42	0.507	0.12	29.43

The complexity results listed also in Table 12 show that the haar filter is the simplest one while the dmey filter is the most complex one. The complexity results show the execution time of the algorithm using any filter normalized to that using the haar filter.

4.2.1. Comparison with FFT-Based Spectral Analysis

Frequency-domain measurements using Fourier analysis calculate the power of selected frequencies within a given frequency range (e.g. the parasympathetic (HF) and sympathetic (LF) frequency ranges). Such conventional spectral analysis methods, although sensitive for extracting information regarding sympathetic and parasympathetic tone, are limited by their inability to adequately assess transient changes in heart rate, which are associated with rapid changes in physiological status [29]. Biological rhythmic behavior such as a heartbeat is non stationary in nature. Thus to be maximally effective, heart rate variability analysis needs to be conducted using non-stationary signal analysis algorithm rather than conventional Fourier analysis.

In [30], a group of 17 patients was identified with diagnosed CHF who had previously had 24 hour Holter monitoring studies as out patients. The Holter tapes were rescanned and examined by Fourier transform. Spectral analysis failed to show significant differences from previously scanned normal subjects.

In [31], the variability of HR and respiratory signals, were analyzed with power spectral analysis to evaluate autonomic control in 25 patients with CHF and 21 normal control subjects. In the CHF patients, HR spectral power was markedly reduced at LF and HF regions. No classification results are included.

The Fourier transform may have a technical limitation in that an underlying periodicity in the data is assumed, whereas the heart rate variability signal is a pseudorandom phenomenon [32].

Wavelet analysis is attractive because it mitigates against the non-stationarities and slow variations inherent in the interbeat-interval sequence. Wavelet analysis permits the time and frequency characteristics of a signal to be simultaneously examined [4].

In order to have a clear idea about the performance of the proposed wavelet-based soft-decision technique in comparison with traditional spectral analysis, an FFT-based spectral analysis screening system which is implemented for this purpose, is included. The comparison is made on long-term records on MIT-trial and test data.

The FFT-based spectral analysis identification system is implemented using the following procedure:

3. The power spectral analysis of the total record length of all trial set data is found by squaring the amplitude spectrum obtained using FFT.
4. The power spectral ratio LF/HF is obtained for each data by finding the ratio of the power spectral density of the LF region (0.0033 to 0.15 Hz) to that of the HF region (0.15 to 0.4 Hz).
5. The threshold value between the CHF data and normal data is found using the ROC analysis. The value is found to be 0.75. The values of the sensitivity, specificity, and accuracy obtained are: 93.33 %, 94.44%, and 93.93% respectively.
6. The performance of the FFT-based technique is evaluated on the test data set. The sensitivity, specificity, and accuracy are obtained as: 82.35%, 81.13%, and 81.42%. Figure 17 shows the PSD ratio (LF/HF) of all data in the test set using FFT spectral analysis.

The three distance metrics are also found to be: TMSD (0.3126), NMSD (0.3804), and PMSD (0.1041). The complexity of The FFT based technique is found as 9.74 times that of the soft-decision approach with haar filters. All results show that the wavelet-based soft-decision technique is better than that of the FFT.

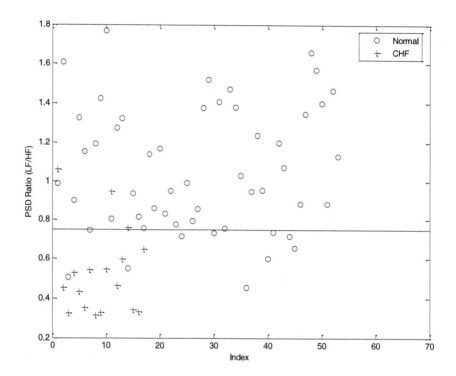

Figure 17. The LF/HF plot for MIT test data using FFT.

4.3. Results of Method 3: Pattern Recognition

4.3.1. Results on Trial and Test Data

Figure 18 and Figure 19 show the values of CF for all CHF and normal data using 32 Sub-bands for trial and test data respectively. The algorithm classifies CHF and normal trial data with an accuracy of 100% (Figure 18) and classifies the test data with sensitivity of (13/17) and with a specificity of (50/53), with an overall identification accuracy of (63/70) 90% (Figure 19).

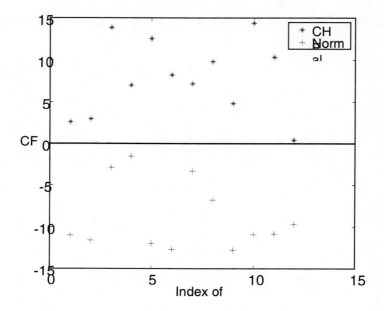

Figure 18. Classification factor results of trial data with 32 sub-bands.

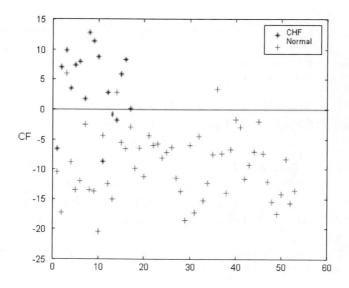

Figure 19. Classification factor results of test data with 32 sub-bands.

4.3.2. Consistency of Results

The leave-one-out method [33] is used to test the consistency of our results. In this method, which is also called partition method, the available set of data (94 records, 24 trial records (12 CHF, 12 normal) and 70 test records (17 CHF, 53 normal)) is divided into $k=n$ subsets which rotate in their use of design (trial) and test. The classifier is designed with n-1 subsets and tested on the remaining subset as follows:

1. Divide the available data into $k=n=5$ subsets (Groups: G1, G2, G3, G4, G5) of randomly patterns. Each subset contains 19 records (6 CHF and 13 normal). G3 contains one CHF data less than other groups.
2. Design the classifier using the first n-1$=4$ subsets and test it on the remaining subset. Estimate the performance of the classifier.
3. Repeat the previous step rotating the position of the test subset, obtaining there by $k=5$ estimates.

Table 13 shows the results of applying this method on 32 sub-bands. This proves that the results obtained on test data are very consistent.

Table 13. Results of leave-one-out-method using 32 sub-bands

Test Group	Sensitivity	Specificity	Accuracy
G1	5/6	10/13	15/19
G2	4/6	11/13	15/19
G3	5/5	11/13	16/18
G4	5/6	13/13	18/19
G5	4/6	11/13	15/19

This method was also tested with 16-subband wavelet decomposition. The accuracy result was almost the same with the 32 subband decomposition. For further investigation of the screening capability, three different distance metrics were used:

PRNMSD: Pattern Recognition Negative Mean Square Distance, which measures the mean square distance of the negative outputs (normal) from the threshold (zero) and is defined as:

$$PRNMSD = \sum_{i=1}^{i=53} CF^2 / 53 \qquad\qquad (28)$$

PRPMSD: Pattern Recognition Positive Mean Square Distance, which
measures the mean square distance of the positive outputs (CHF) from
the threshold (zero) and is defined as:

$$PRPMSD = \sum_{i=1}^{i=17} CF^2 / 17 \qquad\qquad (29)$$

PRTMSD: Pattern Recognition Total Mean Square Distance, which
measures the mean square distance of all outputs (normal and CHF)
from the threshold (zero) and is defined as:

$$PRTMSD = \sum_{i=1}^{i=70} CF^2 / 70 \qquad\qquad (30)$$

Where CF is the classification factor for 53 (normal) and 17 (CHF) test
data.These distance metrics are listed in Table 14. From this table, it can be
concluded that increasing the sub-bands from 16 to 32, improves the results
(the distances of classified points from threshold).

Table 14. Distance metrics for different subbands

Sub-bands	PRTMSD	PRNMSD	PRPMSD
16	14.49	15.17	12.38
32	108.85	121.91	58.65

The pattern recognition method results in identical accuracy values when
it is used with 16 or 32 sub-bands, while the consistency of the method is
improved as the number of sub-bands increases from 16 to 32. On the other
hand the complexity of the algorithm is increased as the number of sub-bands
increases from 16 to 32 sub-bands. It has been found that the execution time of
the complete program of obtaining the pattern of the signal under test and
compare it with both standard patterns and finding the result of identification
of the subject, is almost doubled when the number of sub-bands increases from
16 to 32, while the time needed only for comparison with both standard

patterns and finding the results of identification is almost the same as the number of sub-bands increases from 16 to 32.

4.3.3. Comparison with Other Techniques

An Accuracy of 100% is achieved in [4] on the same trial data at window scales of 16-samples and 32-samples using some individual wavelets parameters. The test data in our study was also investigated in a time-domain technique in [6], which resulted in an accuracy of 93.2%. Both techniques in [4] and [6] can not be considered as screening techniques because neither of them was implemented on both trial and test data. So their results can be considered as data-dependent. The same drawback is applied on our work in [14]. Since the 100% efficiency was obtained only on trial data.

On the opposite, our proposed technique in this section is implemented on both trial data and test data with an accuracy of 100% and 90% respectively and with a total accuracy of 92.55%. Two average standard plots are obtained from trial data and then have been used to identify the test data.

5. CONCLUSION

Non-invasive diagnosis techniques based on analysis of RRI data for screening of patients with congestive heart failure are much required in hospitals and preferred by both doctors and patients due to their simplicity. Three non-invasive techniques are investigated in this chapter for diagnosis of CHF from normal subjects.

SSC is a time domain analysis method that has been utilized newly in this work to discriminate between CHF and NSR records. Two RRI data groups were used; one as trial group and the other as test group. The SSC was applied to three window lengths of the amplitude and frequency attributes of the RRI data that are produced by the Hilbert transform. The three windows are: 16-samples, 32-samples and 300-samples. Out of the eight SSC parameters, only three parameters produced reliable results. By using a single SSC parameter, an accuracy of 96.97% was obtained on amplitude attributes of the trial data at different window lengths, and accuracy of 92.9% was obtained on the test data. A voting process was used between the three selected parameters to produce the final classification. Voting produced maximum accuracy of 93.9% on trial data and 92.9% on test data. The results of this study are consistent to [4] where higher separation between NSR and CHF subject was made at scale of 16 samples and 32 samples. In this study, reliable discrimination was also achieved at scales of 300-samples.

Different wavelet-decomposition filters were used with a soft-decision algorithm for estimating the approximate power spectral density of RRI data for the purpose of screening CHF patients from normal subjects. The power ratio of the LF band to that of the HF band is used as classification factor. The CHF subjects are found to exhibit less HRV (lower power) than normal subjects in the low frequency band. The threshold value of the classification factor is obtained using ROC on 33 MIT trial data. The selected threshold value is then used to screen the 70 MIT test data. The best results obtained for MIT trial data are: specificity of 94.44%, sensitivity of 93.3% and accuracy of 93.93%. The results for MIT test data are: specificity of 90.6%, sensitivity of 82.4%, accuracy of 88.6%. The different wavelet filters are compared in terms of complexity and distance metrics.

A complete FFT-based screening system is also implemented on the same data for comparison. The wavelet-based soft-decision results are shown to be better than that of FFT. In general, the dmey wavelet results are the best with an accuracy of 88.6% obtained by soft-decision on the whole record.

A soft decision algorithm of PSD estimation of decomposed wavelet sub-bands is implemented to obtain two standard plots of CHF and normal subject for the purpose of classification between them in a new pattern recognition method. The base-2 logarithmic values of the reciprocal of the estimated PSD (with db4 wavelets) have been used to compute the classification factor. The power spectral density of the HRV of CHF patients is reduced compared to that of normal subject especially at LF region. The frequency range (0.0625 to 0.4375) Hz of the PSD spectrum of the RRI data is used in the recognition. An accuracy of 100% is obtained on 24 MIT trail data and 90% on 70 MIT test data.

In heart failure progression, the total power as well as the power of LF components is progressively reduced. LF and HF spectral components could be the prominent parameters for discriminating between the different stages of heart failure. Such idea could be used to promote HRV as a monitoring technique in heart failure treatment. Further research in this area is to monitor whether medical treatment can increase the reduced HRV in CHF patients.

REFERENCES

[1] Heart Failure Society of America, Questions About HF [online]. Available: www.abouthf.org

[2] Task Force of the European Society of Cardiology and the North American Society of Pacing and Electrophysiology, Heart rate variability, standards of measurements, physiological interpretation, and clinical use, *Circulation* 93, pp. 1043-1065, 1996.

[3] Ponikowski, P., Anker S.D., Chau T.P. et al; Depressed heart rate variability as an independent predictor of death in chronic congestive heart failure secondary to ischemic or idiopathic dialeted cardiomyopathy. *AM J. Cardio.*, 79, 1645-1650, 1997.

[4] M. C. Teich, S. B. Lowen, B. M. Jost, K. Vibe-Rheymer, and C. Heneghan, "Heart Rate Variability: Measures and Models," in *Nonlinear Biomedical Signal Processing*, Vol. II, *Dynamic Analysis and Modeling*, edited by M. Akay (IEEE Press, New York, 2001), ch. 6, pp. 159-213;

[5] B. Reiner, H-W. Martin, N. Jorg and P. Thomas," Heart rate Variability in infants with heart failure due to congenital heart disease: reversal of depressed heart rate variability by propranolol," *Med. Sci Monit*, 8(10): pp. 661-666, 2002. Available: *http://www.MedSciMonit.com/pub/vol_8/no_10/2875.pdf*

[6] M. H. Asyali, "Discrimination power of long-term heart rate variability measures, "*Proceedings of the 25th Annual International Conference of the IEEE*, Vol. 1,PP.200-203, Sept. 2003.

[7] J. E. Mietus, C-K Peng, I Henry, R. L. Goldsmith and A. L. Goldberger," The pNNx files: re-examining a widely used heart rate variability measure," *Heart*, 88, pp.378-380, 2002.

[8] Al Ghunaimi, A. Hossen, M. O. Hassan," Statistical Signal Characterization for Congestive Heart Failure Patient's Classification", *Technology and Health Care Journal*,Vol. 14, No.1, pp.29-45, 2006.

[9] B. Al Ghunaimi, A. Hossen, and M. O. Hassan, "Screening of obstructive sleep apnea based on statistical signal characterization of Hilbert transform of RRI data," *Technology and Health Care*, 12 (1), pp.67-78, 2004.

[10] A. Hossen and B. Al Ghunaimi, "A Wavelet-Based Soft Decision Technique for Patients with Congestive Heart Failure Patient Classification", *Biomedical Signal Processing and Control*, 2, pp. 135-143, 2007.

[11] A. Hossen, A soft decision algorithm for obstructive sleep apnea patient classification based on fast estimation of wavelet entropy of RRI data, Technology and Health care;3, pp. 151-165, 2005.

[12] A. Hossen, B. Al-Ghunaimi, and M.O. Hassan, A new simple algorithm for heart rate variability analysis in patients with obstructive sleep apnea and normal controls, *International Journal of Bioelectromagnetism,* 5(1), pp. 238-239, 2003.

[13] A. Hossen, B. Al-Ghunaimi, M.O Hassan, Subband decomposition soft decision algorithm for heart rate variability analysis in patients with OSA and normal controls, *Signal Processing*; 85, pp. 95-106, 2005.

[14] A. Hossen, B. Al-Ghunaimi, A new method for screening of patients with congestive heart failure, *International Journal of Computational Intelligence,* 1(3):266-270, 2004.

[15] A. Hossen, Power spectral density estimation via wavelet decomposition, *Electronics Letters*, 40(17), pp. 1055-1056, 2004.

[16] PhysioNet: An NIH/NCRR Research Resource for Complex Physiologic Signals, apnea-ecg [data files online]. Available: http://www.physionet.org/physiobank/database/

[17] PhysioNet: An NIH/NCRR Research Resource for Complex Physiologic Signals, The WFDB software package. [online]. Available: http://www.physionet.org/physiotools/wfdb.shtml

[18] Jr. Thomas, Overview of RR variability, Heart Rhythm Instruments Inc, 2002 [Cited 2003 Jun 02]. Available from: http://www.nervexpress.com/overview.html

[19] G. M. Friesen, T. C. Jannett, M. A. Jadallah, et al, "A Comparison of the noise sensitivity of nine QRS detection algorithms," *IEEE Trans. Biomed. Eng.* 37(1), pp.85-97, Jan., 1990.

[20] J. E. Mietus, C. K. Peng, P. Ch. Ivanov, and A. L. Goldberger, "Detection of obstructive sleep apnea from cardiac interbeat interval time series," *Computers in Cardiology.* [online]. Vol. 27, pp. 753-756, 2000. Available: http://www.physionet.org/physiotools/apdet/apdet.shtml

[21] S. K. Mitra, Digital Signal Processing: A computer-Based Approach, 2nd ed., McGraw-Hill International Edition, NY, pp.794-765, 2002.

[22] M. S. Roden, *Analog and Digital Communication System*, 3ed ed., Prentice Hall International Edition, N.J, p. 235, 1991.

[23] H. L. Hirsch, *Statistical Signal Characterization*. USA: Artech House Inc., pp. 25-27, 1992.

[24] A. Hossen, and U. Heute, Fully Adaptive Evaluation of SB-DFT, *Proceedings of IEEE Int. Symp. on Circuits and Systems*, Chicago, Illinois, 1993.

[25] R. M. Rangayyan, *Biomedical Signal Analysis: A Case-Study Approach,* John Wiley & Sons, Inc., U.S.A., pp.466-472, Dec., 2001.

[26] O. Aleksander, Discernibility and Rough Sets in Medicine: Tools and Applications [M.S Thesis online]. Norway: Norwegian University of Science and Technology, pp.71-81. [Cited Dec 16, 1999]. Available from: www.idi.ntnu.no/~aleks/thesis/main.ps

[27] F. Provost, T. Fawcett, "Robust classification for imprecise environments," *Machine Learning*, vol. 42, pp. 203- 231, 2000.

[28] A. Hossen, B. Al Ghunaimi, "A Pattern recognition technique based on wavelet decomposition for identification of patients with congestive heart failure", TJER, Vol. 6, No. 2, 2009, pp.40-46.

[29] Drs. Irving, F. Miller, D. B. Yeates, L. B. Wong, Heart Rate Variability Analysis – Promise and Fulfillment, A Report in Business Briefing, Global Healthcare, *Advanced Medical Technologies,* pp. 1-4, 2004.

[30] M. Majercik, C.L. Bull, Analysis of heart rate variability by Fourier analysis in a group of patients diagnosed with congestive heart failure, *Proceedings of the Annual Conference on Engineering in Medicine and Biology,* 13, pp. 676-678, 1991.

[31] J. P. Saul, Y. Arai, R. D. Berger, L. S. Lilly. W. S. Colucci, and R. J. Cohen, Assessment of autonomic regulation in chronic congestive heart failure by heart rate spectral analysis, *The American Journal of cardiology*, 61(15), pp. 1292-1299, 1988.

[32] F. Notarius, J.S. Floras, Limitations of the use of spectral analysis of heart rate variability for the estimation of cardiac sympathetic activity in heart failure, *Europace*, 3(1), pp. 29-38, 2001.

[33] J.P. Marques de Sa, Pattern Recognition, Concepts, Methods and Applications, Springer Verlag, 2002.

INDEX

B

E

I

J

K

L

M

Q

T

U

V